# Delirium in Elderly Patients

Ahmet Turan Isik • George T. Grossberg
Editors

# Delirium in Elderly Patients

Springer

*Editors*
Ahmet Turan Isik
Department of Geriatric Medicine
Dokuz Eylul University
School of Medicine
Izmir
Turkey

George T. Grossberg
Department of Neurology and Psychiatry
Saint Louis University
School of Medicine
St. Louis, Missouri
USA

ISBN 978-3-319-65237-5 ISBN 978-3-319-65239-9 (eBook)
https://doi.org/10.1007/978-3-319-65239-9

Library of Congress Control Number: 2017960952



Printed on acid-free paper

This Springer imprint is published by Springer Nature
The registered company is Springer International Publishing AG
The registered company address is: Gewerbestrasse 11, 6330 Cham, Switzerland

# Preface

Delirium is a cognitive disorder characterized by deficits in attention, arousal, consciousness, memory, orientation, perception, speech, and language. It is a common and serious problem among older persons at every healthcare interface. Despite its importance in terms of clinical, economic, and social considerations, and despite considerable advances up to now, it remains a relatively misunderstood and misdiagnosed condition. A formal cognitive assessment as well as a history of acute onset of symptoms is necessary for the diagnosis of delirium. In addition, delirium is evaluated as a geriatric medical emergency until proven otherwise, in geriatric practice.

*Delirium in Elderly patients* provides a comprehensive, scholarly, and practical account of delirium for all doctors and nurses involved in the care of the elderly. This book not only provides a state-of-the-art update on delirium covering its history, epidemiology, pathophysiology, assessment, diagnosis, causes, prevention, and management but also provides evidence-based and practical information related to delirium for daily geriatric practice. In addition, due to the complex multifactorial causes of delirium, different aspects of delirium in the elderly are discussed from a variety of perspectives, including geriatrician, geriatric psychiatrist, neurologist, intensive care specialist, and nursing, in this book. At the end, the case vignettes, the scale related to the delirium, and the list of those drugs highly associated with delirium enhance the value of the book.

This book will be of interest to professionals working in geriatrics, geriatric psychiatry, general psychiatry, or neurology as well as internist, intensive care unit specialist, and all those who care for the elderly in hospitals or the community.

We wish to express our appreciation for the efforts of all the dedicated scientists who provided their experience in this book.

Izmir, Turkey — Ahmet Turan Isik
St. Louis, MO — George T. Grossberg

The original version of the book was revised. "Appendix: Delirium Assessment Instruments" has been included in the backmatter of the book. The correction to the book is available at https://doi.org/10.1007/978-3-319-65239-9_12.

# Contents

# Delirium: From Past to Present

1

Derya Kaya

Delirium is one of the most common seen mental illnesses that is mainly characterized with a disturbance in attention or change in cognition. It has particularly a long description history beginning from ancient and medieval times up to the nineteenth century (Goodrick, 2015). Studies toward understanding of its pathophysiology take place during the twentieth century.

Dating back to the works of Hippocrates (460–366 B.C.), without naming "delirium" and mental abnormalities due to fever, poisons, or head trauma, the word "phrenitis" was used, and also the word "lethargus" was introduced for stating inertia and dulling of the senses (Lipourlis, 1983). Indeed, two main variants of delirium, a restlessness, insomniac, hallucinogenic state and, the other form, a lethargic and sleepiness state, violent and low according to Lipowski (1990), the so-called hypoactive and hyperactive delirium today, were described by Hippocrates, too (Lipowski 1990). The term "delirium," deriving from the Latin "deliro-delirare" and meaning "offtrack," was accepted to be firstly used by Celsus in the first century A.D. (Celsus 1935). Celsus was also known to report for the first time that nonfebrile causes could be the reason for the development of delirium (Adamis et al. 2007). In the second century, the Cappadocian medical writer, Aretaeus, remarked that delirium differed from chronic illnesses (dementia) in terms of duration and was probably the first who recommended a quiet and dark room for a delirious patient and hasheesh (boiled poppy) (Adams 1861). Other medical writers of the same century, Soranus (A.D. 93–138) and Galen (A.D. 131–200), had also put forward therapeutic approaches that are still feasible today. The importance of ensuring sleep was emphasized by Soranus, and the requirement of finding and treating the underlying condition affecting the brain was firstly stressed by Galen (Lipowski 1990). As Lipowski (1991), the father of delirium history, stressed, defending an

D. Kaya, M.D.
Unit for Brain Aging and Dementia, Faculty of Medicine, Department of Geriatric Medicine, Dokuz Eylul University, 35340 Izmir, Turkey
e-mail: deryakaya29@gmail.com



A.T. Isik, G.T. Grossberg (eds.), *Delirium in Elderly Patients*,
https://doi.org/10.1007/978-3-319-65239-9_1

organic underlying cause and nonpharmacological treatment approaches in the same century was a very noteworthy fact.

Although it seems like the flow of the history of the disorder keeps on track till these lines, it should be underlined that the meaning of delirium was full of confusing relevant terminology throughout for many centuries, such as mania with fever, acute mental insanity, clouding of consciousness, and epileptic excitement (Caraceni and Grassi 2011; Lipowski 1991). The unchanging presence of fever; the difficulties in distinguishing from such chronic conditions as mania, psychoses, and dementia; and the presence of both primary and secondary causes were providing the main basis for the terminological descriptive ambiguity.

The core clinical features of delirium were specified in detail in the English medical literature in Philip Barrough's textbook (*The Method of Physick*, 1583). The disturbances in cognition, in memory, in imagination, and in sleep were involved as the main features of the disorder. Later on the sixteenth and seventeenth centuries, an increasing number of publications on this mental disorder had appeared. In one of them, in Thomas Willis' publication (1683), the disorder was regarded as a symptom rather than a disease, could result from the state of being drunk, and included impaired global cognitive status, sleep, perception, and psychomotor behavior (Lipowski 1991; Willis 1683). In the course of time, disturbed sleep has attracted attention, so that it was reported that the disorder resembled a sort of waking dream from disordered sleep (Hunter 1835). Today as disrupted sleep-wake cycle is considered to be frequently affected in delirium, melatonin and a melatonin agonist, ramelteon, are being studied in prevention and treatment studies of delirium (Al-Aama et al. 2011; Sultan 2010). The first treatise with regard to delirium in English was reported to be published by Frings in the eighteenth century (Frings 1746). It was also only in the eighteenth century that delirium was well defined different from mania and melancholia (Sims 1799).

In the nineteenth century coming to an end to defining delirium with various terms, medical writers began to focus on the psychopathology of the disorder. Impaired consciousness, clouding of consciousness, was linked to delirium (Greiner 1817). Delirium tremens was introduced as a distinct entity. The concept of clouding of consciousness had been evolved in the 1860s explaining consciousness in delirium is a widely varying spectrum from a slight confusion to coma that resulted from dissolution of the highest parts of the nervous system and so disinhibition of the evolutionally lower parts (Lipowski 1991). One of the clinical hallmarks of the disorder, waxing and waning, was spelled out. The nineteenth century was the century of focusing efforts to use "clouding of consciousness" as a separator for delirium. Likewise, "confusion" and then "acute confusional state" (Lipowski 1990) were derived as an alternative separator for the differential diagnosis (Lindesay 1999); however, all these three terms were reported to be seen in some other conditions such as catatonic stupor, transient hysterical state, or when using ecstasy (Lipowski 1990). On the other hand, clouding of consciousness was involved into Diagnostic and Statistical Manual of Mental Disorders (DSM)-III delirium criteria, the first diagnostic criteria developed by an expert committee, but this concept was omitted in DSM-III-R (American Psychiatric Association 1987) for being difficult to measure. Nevertheless, the notion of delirium was settled as an acute transient cognitive impairment; disturbed attention, with fluctuating consciousness and disturbed perception; and delusions by the late nineteenth century.

In the beginning of twentieth century, Bonhoeffer was the one who considered clouding of consciousness as the main figure of delirium and grouped delirium as one of the five "acute exogenous reaction types" (Bonhoeffer 1912) which meant acute mental manifestations observed secondarily because of systemic diseases. His view provided further modern aspects for latter psychiatric syndromes related to physical illnesses. Later in 1935, Wolff and Curran held this reaction type as "dysergastic reaction" in the psychiatric perspective (Wolff and Curran 1935). One of the most remarkable developments in the concept of delirium was performed by Engel and Romano in 1940s (Engel and Romano 1959). They performed EEG work and concluded that delirium was a cognitive and attentional disorder affecting the level of consciousness that resulted from the reduction of the cerebral metabolic rate which was correlated with the slowing of the EEG background activity. In regard of this accelerative observation, not only an innovative laboratory parameter was gained but also a link between pathophysiological and the psychological variables. Later by Blass et al., this pathophysiological hypothesis moved to the presence of decreased neurotransmitter synthesis, particularly acetylcholine, due to disturbed oxidative metabolism as existed in the metabolic encephalopathies (Blass et al. 1981). Additionally, occurrence of delirium was achieved further by administering anticholinergic drugs (Lipowski 1990). This and former clinical and experimental studies on cholinergic blockade led to a new era in the pathogenic approach of delirium and probably the first for delirium superimposed on Alzheimer's dementia, the so-called central cholinergic deficiency, that is, also prevailed as an important landmark in Alzheimer's dementia (Cummings and Benson 1987).

Throughout all these courses of time and studies, a need to cross talk, to collaborative research, and to teach had emerged so that diagnostic criteria have been formulated by expert committees. While acute organic brain syndrome had been used to refer delirium till late twentieth century (Lipowski 1980), with recommendation of Lipowski ZJ, the term "delirium" was decided to be involved into the classifications. The diagnostic criteria for delirium have been formulated in two main classification systems, the first one is of American Psychiatric Association, DSM, and the latter is of "International Classification of Diseases" (ICD) in the last part of the twentieth century. The line of the core clinical features and diagnostic criteria for delirium had drawn in DSM-III (American Psychiatric Association 1980). Dropping the concept of organic mental disorder existed in DSM-III, DSM-IV was published. It provided widely used definitions, and the disorder has been regarded an acute and fluctuating cerebral dysfunction that was not better accounted for a preexisting, established, or evolving dementia and existed as disturbance of consciousness, especially attention, and change in cognition (memory, orientation, language, perception). Direct evidence must be established from the history of the patients or the physical examination or laboratory findings that symptoms are physiological consequences due to a general medical problem (American Psychiatric Association 2000). International Classification of Diseases-10 resembles DSM-IV with some exceptions such that it still involves the concept of organic brain disorder (World Health Organization 1993). This classification has been criticized for being insufficient for researchers due to lack of sensitivity to correctly identify true cases of delirium. With a less degree of problem, DSM-IV has also been criticized for some reasons. The need of adequate assessment of attention particularly in the hypoactive period, more detailed characterization of some neuropsychological features such as thought process abnormalities, and sleep-wake cycle, and defining clinical subtypes, as well as duration, course, and severity of the disorder, are some of the focused criticized points (Caraceni and Grassi 2011). Finally, the criteria have been updated in DSM-V (American Psychiatric Association 2013), and delirium is defined as a disturbance in attention and awareness, developing over a short period of time, typically hours to days with a change in baseline attention and awareness, and it fluctuates throughout the day. Disturbance in cognition such as in memory, orientation, language, and perception should exist, and the two disturbances should not be better explained by another neurocognitive disorder. And as in DSM-IV, there must also be evidence that the delirium is due to a direct physiological consequence of another medical condition, substance intoxication or withdrawal, or exposure to a toxin or is due to multiple etiologies (American Psychiatric Association 2013).

There would be probably cases that could not be defined as delirium according to the classification systems. In the pages of history, delirium was and still is a clinical diagnosis, and this could be the best explanation of the continuum between delirium and "normality." To conclude, there are undeniable universal realities that come from ancient times such that delirium is a global cognitive impairment due to cholinergic insufficiency, associated with poor mortality and morbidity; is more persistent than previously believed, unfortunately underdiagnosed but treatable if diagnosed early and managed properly; and has deleterious effects on long-term cognitive functioning in elderly patients with dementia, and lastly the real underlying medical conditions should be identified.

## References

Adamis D, A Treloar A, FC Martin FC et al (2007) A brief review of the history of delirium as a mental disorder. Hist Psychiatry 18:459–469

Adams F (1861) The extant works of Aretaeus. In: Adams F (ed) The Cappadocian. Sydenham Society, London

Al-Aama T, Brymer C, Gutmanis I et al (2011) Melatonin decreases delirium in elderly patients: a randomized, placebo-controlled trial. Int J Geriatr Psychiatry 26:687–694

American Psychiatric Association (1980) Diagnostic and statistical manual of mental disorders 3rd ed. American Psychiatric Association, Washington, DC

American Psychiatric Association (1987) Diagnostic and statistical manual of mental disorders III-R text revision. American Psychiatric Association, Washington, DC

American Psychiatric Association (2000) Diagnostic and statistical manual of mental disorders 4th ed. American Psychiatric Association, Washington, DC

American Psychiatric Association (2013) Diagnostic and statistical manual of mental disorders 5th ed. American Psychiatric Association, Washington, DC

Barrough P (1583) The method of Physick. Field, London
Blass JP, Gibson GE, Duffy TE et al (1981) Cholinergic dysfunction: a common denominator in metabolic encephalopathies. In: Pepeu G, Ladinsky H (eds) Cholinergic mechanisms. Plenum Press, New York
Bonhoeffer K (1912) Die Psychosen im Gefolge von akuten Infektionen, Allgemeinerkrankungen und inneren Erkrankungen. In: Aschaffenburg GL (ed) Handbuch der psychiatrie. Deuticke, Leipzig
Caraceni A, Grassi L (2011) Delirium acute confusional state in palliative medicine, 2nd edn. Oxford University Press, Oxford
Celsus (1935) On medicine. Books I–IV (trans: Spencer WG). Harvard University Press, Cambridge, MA
Cummings JL, Benson DF (1987) The role of the nucleus basalis of Meynert in dementia: review and reconsideration. Alzheimer Dis Assoc Disord 1:128–145
Engel GL, Romano J (1959) Delirium, a syndrome of cerebral insufficiency. J Chronic Dis 9:260–277
Frings P (1746) A treatise on phrensy. Gardner, London
Goodrick S (2015) The hinterland of delirium. Lancet Neurol 14(8):792
Greiner GFC (1817) Der Traum und das fi eberhafte Irreseyn. Ein physiologisch psychologischer Versuch. F. A. Brockhaus, Altenburg und Leipzig
Hunter J (1835) In: Palmer JF (ed) The work of John Hunter, FRS, vol 1. Longman, London
Lindesay J (1999) The concept of delirium. Dement Geriatr Cogn Disord 10:310–314
Lipourlis D (1983) Ιπποκρατικη Ιατρικη [Hippocratic Medicine]. Paratiritis, Thessalonika
Lipowski ZJ (1980) A new look at the organic brain syndromes. Am J Psychiatry 137:674–678
Lipowski ZJ (1990) Delirium: acute confusional state. Oxford University, New York
Lipowski ZL (1991) Delirium: how its concept has developed. Int Psychogeriatr 3:115–120
Sims J (1799) Pathological remarks upon various kinds of alienation of mind. Mem R Soc Lond 5:372–406
Sultan SS (2010) Assessment of role of perioperative melatonin in prevention and treatment of postoperative delirium after hip arthroplasty under spinal anesthesia in the elderly. Saudi J Anaesth 4:169–173
Willis T (1683) Two discourses concerning the soul of brutes. Bring, Harper and Leigh, London
Wolff HG, Curran D (1935) Nature of delirium and allied states: the dysergastic reaction. Arch Neurol Psychiatr 33:1175–1215
World Health Organization (1993) The ICD-10 classification of mental and behavioural disorders. Diagnostic Criteria for Research, World Health Organization, Geneva

# Pathogenesis of Delirium

# 2

Pinar Soysal and Ahmet Turan Isik

Considering physiopathological processes of delirium, it is possible to see that numerous precipitating and predisposing factors, each of which would facilitate development of delirium, are interacting with each other in the majority of cases. As conventional electrophysiological tests, brain imaging, and neurotransmitter analyses are not always possible in the cases and the results of animal studies do not overlap one to one, physiopathological mechanisms of delirium have not been enlightened yet (Isik 2014).

Diversity of defined risk factors and neurochemical abnormalities suggests that brain dysfunction in delirium results from the interaction among numerous systems. Therefore, it seems impossible to explain delirium by a single etiological theorem. However, evidences that delirium is a neurotoxic picture which develops due primarily to neurotransmitter (cholinergic insufficiency) and inflammatory (increase in stress response/neuroinflammation) mechanisms (Matto et al. 2010) are increasing each passing day (Mac Lullich et al. 2009).

Since the basic problem in the disease is the maintenance of attention, trying to understand the neurobiology of attention would be the best approach (Isik 2014). Normal attention function requires integrity of the ascending reticular activating system (ARAS) in the superior part of the brain stem and polymodal association areas in the cortex. Stimulation of ARAS enables alertness; whereas destruction may cause sleep, coma, and akinetic mutism. ARAS directs the cortex for stimulus uptake; polymodal association areas focus and control the alertness energy necessary for attention. Prefrontal cortex and posterior parietal cortex play an important role in the regulation of attention. Prefrontal cortex primarily enables the maintenance of attention. Risk factors defined for delirium may cause various confusional states by

P. Soysal
Associate Professor, Geriatric Center, Kayseri Education and Training Hospital, Kayseri, Turkey

A.T. Isik (✉)
Unit for Aging Brain and Dementia, Department of Geriatric Medicine, Faculty of Medicine, Dokuz Eylul University, 35340 Izmir, Turkey
e-mail: atisik@yahoo.com



A.T. Isik, G.T. Grossberg (eds.), *Delirium in Elderly Patients*,
https://doi.org/10.1007/978-3-319-65239-9_2

impairing the ascending effect of ARAS and descending control of frontal, parietal, and limbic cortex on attention and/or by influencing regulation of area-specific attention functions (Isik 2009, 2014). Studies on evoked potentials of brain stem and on brain imaging indicate that not only the cortical structures but also subcortical structures such as thalamus, basal ganglia, and pons reticular formation play an important role in the pathogenesis of delirium (Cerejeir et al. 2010). ARAS influences cerebral cortex both directly and by means of thalamic nuclear signals; therefore, delirium may observed even with small lesions in thalamus.

Similar condition can develop in case of dysfunction of basal ganglia, which are responsible for multidirectional connection between thalamus, brain stem, and cerebral cortex. Delirium being more prevalent in basal ganglion diseases such as subcortical stroke and Parkinson's disease supports this hypothesis (Trzepacz 1994; Benbadis et al. 1994).

Chaotic process in delirium is observed not only in the anatomy of the disease but also in the physiopathology just as the same. Therefore, we consider that discussing the mechanisms that focus on in the development of delirium under separate topics would be beneficial.

## 2.1 Dysfunctions Associated with Neurotransmitters

It is thought that documented etiological factors of delirium act over similar mechanisms by altering functions of neuronal membrane and leading to a series of neurotransmitter abnormalities. Probably, delirium results from the interaction between numerous neurotransmitters, mainly acetylcholine and dopamine, and cortical and subcortical pathways. Any situation that influences function, synthesis, and secretion of neurotransmitters can lead to delirium (Mittal et al. 2011).

According to the neurotransmitter hypothesis, etiological factors cause neurotransmitter abnormalities by impairing cerebral oxidative metabolism, and consequently cerebral dysfunction occurs. Decrease in cholinergic activity and increase or decrease in serotonergic and γ-aminobutyrinergic (GABAergic) activity due to oversecretion of dopamine, norepinephrine, and glutamate may be effective in delirium presenting itself with different symptoms (Matto et al. 2010; Van Der Mast 1998).

### 2.1.1 Acetylcholine

It is not surprising that cholinergic system, which is important for attention and cognitive functions, plays a role also in the development of delirium. Current evidences suggest that cholinergic system is effective in the development of delirium. While anticholinergics facilitate development of delirium, severity of delirium clinic is enhanced with the intensity of drug-related anticholinergic activity (Martins and Fernandes 2012). Since acetylcholine (ACh), which is the basic transmitter of cholinergic system, is synthesized from "acetyl coenzyme A" by an ATP-dependent reaction, acetylcholine production is in close association with energy cycle of the neurons. Therefore, cerebral ACh production is influenced by any condition that affects oxidative metabolism such as hypoxia or inflammation. ACh insufficiency that results from neuronal loss in cholinergic system may be a reason for tendency to delirium in dementia cases (Terry and Buccafusco 2003). In brief, neurotransmitter imbalances due to the factors such as ischemia and global stressors and impairment in acetylcholine synthesis and cholinergic synaptic mechanisms lead to cholinergic insufficiency and consequently to delirium, no matter how diverse the etiological factors are (Mittal et al. 2011; Hshieh et al. 2008). Despite the presence of very strong evidences supporting cholinergic insufficiency hypothesis, this hypothesis has weaknesses. For example, benefits of cholinesterase inhibitors in the treatment of delirium are limited. Moreover, why clinical presentation of Alzheimer disease and delirium is different (attention disorder in delirium, memory disorder in Alzheimer disease) although they are physiopathologically associated with each other cannot be explained completely (Hshieh et al. 2008). On the other hand, that patients with postoperative delirium have lower plasma cholinesterase levels in the preoperative period has brought potential to the acetyl and butyrylcholinesterase enzymes for being biomarkers of postoperative delirium. This result may explain why cholinesterase inhibitors are not as much effective as expected in the treatment of delirium (Cerejeira and Mukaetova-Ladinska 2011).

### 2.1.2 Dopamine

Acetylcholine hypothesis should be considered together with dopamine hypothesis as they have close relationship in the brain. The conditions with increased dopamine levels cause development of delirium. Dopamine is effective in the occurrence of delirium clinic, primarily of the psychotic symptoms, by playing a role in motor activity and cognitive functions such as attention, thinking, and perception (Van Der Mast 1998). Dopamine blockers are used in the treatment of delirium until the underlying causes are improved as they help temporary balance of acetylcholinergic and dopaminergic activities. These drugs provide temporary improvement until underlying reasons are improved (Mittal et al. 2011). Studies demonstrated that dopamine antagonists caused motor hyperactivity similar to that in hyperactive delirium and EEG revealed low wave pattern. Increased dopamine usually causes appearance of the symptoms such as increase in psychomotor activity, irritability, agitation, disturbance, aggressiveness, and psychosis (Maldonado 2008).

Although the effects of the other neurotransmitters such as GABA, serotonin (5-hydroxytryptamine [5HT]), and norepinephrine have not been as well documented as that of acetylcholine and dopamine, their contribution to the development of delirium is known (Mittal et al. 2011).

### 2.1.3 Serotonin

Serotonin (5HT) is an important neurotransmitter in the development of delirium in both surgical and medical patients. Synthesis and secretion of 5HT in the brain depend on the presence of tryptophan, which is the precursor of 5HT (Maldonado 2008). Increase and decrease in serotonergic activity are effective in the development of delirium. It is determined that serotonergic activity is particularly decreased in hyperactive delirium and increased in hypoactive delirium. Human and animal studies demonstrate that serotonin concentrations increased in hepatic encephalopathy and septic delirium (White 2002). Extremely increased serotonergic activity causes occurrence of psychotic symptoms, which are among the basic symptoms of serotonergic syndrome and delirium. On the other hand, decrease in cerebral tryptophan level and accordingly decrease in serotonergic functions have been determined in delirium tremens. Therefore, neuropsychiatric symptoms just like in delirium clinic are quite common in conditions which selective serotonin reuptake inhibitors are withdrawn too quickly (Maldonado 2008).

### 2.1.4 Gamma-Aminobutyric Acid

Gamma-aminobutyric acid (GABA) is the main inhibitor neurotransmitter of the central nervous system (CNS). Agents like propofol and benzodiazepines, which are frequently used in hospitals and intensive care units, show high affinity to GABAergic receptors, particularly in the brain stem. Cerebral functional integrity is impaired, and maintenance of alertness becomes difficult as the result of excessive neurotransmission in the CNS (Maldonado 2008). While GABA activity is increased in hepatic encephalopathy, it is decreased in delirium due to barbiturate withdrawing (Weinberger 1993). Increase in ammonium concentration in the patients with hepatic encephalopathy causes increase in glutamate and glutamine, which are the precursors of GABA. Hyperactivity of locus coeruleus and its noradrenergic neurons is in question in delirium due to alcohol withdrawing (White 2002).

### 2.1.5 Glutamate

Glutamate is the neurotransmitter of N-methyl-D-aspartate (NMDA) receptors in the CNS. Ischemic injury allows $Ca^{+2}$ transport into the cell and accordingly causes significant increase in extracellular glutamate levels and glutamate receptor activation. Excitatory glutamate that is increased under hypoxic conditions activates NMDA receptors and may cause neuronal injury. Nevertheless, dopamine is required for glutamate toxicity, which is also known as $Ca^{+2}$-related neurotoxicity. When dopamine reaches to high levels, it may enhance excitatory effect of glutamate by causing adequate neuron depolarization for the activation of voltage-dependent NMDA receptors. Overstimulation of NMDA receptors as well causes neuronal injury and death (Maldonado 2008).

## 2.2 Inflammatory Response

Delirium can accompany many medical and surgical conditions with increased inflammatory response. Therefore, delirium may manifest itself sometimes as a condition that accompany sepsis-related multi-organ failure (Siami et al. 2008), sometimes as a presenting clinic of underlying simple urinary system infection or pneumonia (particularly in elder dementia patients) and sometimes as a postoperative complication (O'Keeffe and Chonchubhair 1994).

### 2.2.1 Cytokines

Systemic inflammatory processes are associated not only with delirium but also with more remarkable neuropsychiatric symptoms. Neuropsychiatric symptoms similar to delirium have been defined long time ago in the patients treated with recombinant IFN (Malek-Ahmadi and Hilsabeck 2007; Cole et al. 2003). Bacterial endotoxin has dose-dependent effect on cognitive functions, emotional state, and sleep in healthy volunteers (Mullington et al. 2000; Reichenberg et al. 2001). Circulating cytokines increase even with very low doses of lipopolysaccharides (LPS) (0.2 ng/kg), and this unfavorably influences the declarative memory and psychomotor activities (Krabbe et al. 2005; Brydon et al. 2008).

It is considered that cognitive changes occur in acute systemic inflammation due to impaired cellular and molecular synergistic relationships in different regions of the brain especially in hippocampus (Tizard 2008). It is known that proinflammatory IL-1 has an important role in neurophysiological processes in memory consolidation probably in the way to regulate synaptic plasticity (Rachal Pugh et al. 2001). IL-6 is effective in hippocampal dysfunction, too (Sparkman et al. 2006). Contrarily, IL-10 balances effects of IL-1 and IL-6, and this seems like to prevent behavioral and cognitive harmful effects of cytokines (Krzyszton et al. 2008; Richwine et al. 2009). In delirium, decrease in the expression of hippocampal brain-derived growth factor (BDGF) and increase in mitochondrial dysfunction and oxidative stress are effective in neuroinflammation that cause learning and memory defects (Noble et al. 2007, Tanaka et al. 2006). All of this information suggests that local cerebral reactive oxygen species (ROS), proinflammatory cytokines, metalloproteinases, nitric oxide, and chemokines can impair learning and memory processes by influencing synaptic plasticity and long-term potentiation processes (McAfoose and Baune 2009).

It has been reported that microglia and astrocyte activation after peripheral immune response may lead to Bax/Bcl-2 imbalance and may influence survival of intraparenchymal brain cell (Semmler et al. 2005). Sharshar et al. (2003) reported that septic shock is associated with neuronal and glial apoptosis within the autonomic centers, which is strongly associated with endothelial inducible nitric oxide synthase (iNOS) expression. Lee et al. (2008) also demonstrated that neuroinflammation-associated amyloidogenesis activation might be an important mechanism associated with neurocognitive dysfunction triggered by apoptotic neuronal cell death and systemic immune stimuli. After peripheral immune stimulation, the cascade of events in the central nervous system can influence neuronal vitality even in the long-term period (Qin et al. 2007).

### 2.2.2 Cortisol

Cortisol is an essential hormone for stress response of the body. Stress response of cortisol increases and duration of response is prolonged in senility and neurodegeneration in dementia (Martins and Fernandes 2012). In the studies, it was determined that cortisol increases not only in blood but also in CSF in delirium patients (Mittal et al. 2011). As excessive glucocorticoid secretion negatively influences mood and memory, they are considered to be effective on pathogenesis of delirium particularly in elderly patients. Excessive glucocorticoid also inhibits glucose transport into the neuron and accordingly neuronal energy deficiency emerges. This particularly affects hippocampus functions (Maldonado 2008). This information appears to explain both increased tendency to delirium and occurrence of delirium clinic in acute stress situations accompanied by high cortisol levels (Martins and Fernandes 2012). Moreover, those high plasma levels of many inflammatory markers, especially cortisol and IL-6, detected both before and during delirium support "extreme stress response/neuroinflammation hypothesis." The presence of relation between cholinergic system and innate immune system over cholinergic inflammatory pathway is an interesting point (Tracey 2009). The regulation of extreme stress response and neuroinflammatory pathway would open new horizons for the treatment of delirium in the future (Cerejeira et al. 2011).

## 2.3 Changes in Neuronal Injury and Permeability of Blood-Brain Barrier (BBB)

Trauma, surgical infection, and metabolic and ischemic reasons cause not only direct neuron injury in the brain but also delirium by increasing proinflammatory cytokines or impairing synthesis and secretion of neurotransmitters such as acetylcholine, dopamine, serotonin, and norepinephrine (Hshieh et al. 2008). In addition, systemic diseases that cause BBB injury may also accompany delirium. BBB injury or dysfunction causes the brain to be exposed to the effect of systemic inflammation (Dimitrijevic et al. 2006).

Factors that precipitate delirium both cause neuronal dysfunction or injury by directly influencing the brain and contribute to the development of an exaggerated inflammatory response. Risk factors of delirium intensively stimulate the limbic hypothalamo-pituitary-adrenal axis, cause immune system activation and stress response, and enhance permeability of BBB (Mittal et al. 2011).

Experimental studies demonstrated that peripheral inflammatory stimuli cause functional and molecular changes in BBB. Increase in permeability of BBB due to change in tight connection proteins has been reported in different inflammatory models. Likewise, peripheral LPS injection (the most commonly used model in inflammation) initiates the cascade of events that cause BBB injury in early period, overexpression of adhesion molecules in endothelial cells, and infiltration of blood leukocytes into the brain tissue (Cerejeir et al. 2010; Semmler et al. 2005; Hofer et al. 2008; Nishioku et al. 2009).

Postmortem studies of human brain tissue also determined mild correlation between systemic inflammation and activation of endothelial and perivascular cells (Uchikado et al. 2004). Although it is difficult to demonstrate BBB injury in human, β subunit of S100 protein (S100-β) can be considered as the evidence for increased

BBB permeability (Marchi et al. 2004). Many conditions, such as septic shock and cardiac surgery, are associated with acute systemic inflammation accompany with BBB (Ali et al. 2000; Gao et al. 1999; Nguyen et al. 2006). In such patients, it was demonstrated that increasing serum S100-β protein during delirium episodes could cause BBB injury (van Munster et al. 2010). In addition, detection of leukoencephalopathy on magnetic resonance imaging (MRI) of delirium cases which were in the early stage of septic shock supports BBB injury (Sharshar et al. 2007). In addition to systemic inflammation, other factors, such as microscopic structure and function, are influenced by hypoxia, ischemia, and pain (McCaffrey et al. 2009; Oztas et al. 2004).

*IGF-I*: Insulin-like growth factor I (IGF-I) is one of the proteins that play a role in the development of human body and in the regulation of various metabolic and brain functions. IGF-I levels decrease with age. IGF-I has an effective role in the development of BBB, neuronal excitability, synthesis of myelin sheath, blood vessel maturation, neuronal vitality, proliferation, differentiation, synaptogenesis, and transport and metabolism of cerebral glucose. IGF-I plays supporting role on neuronal plasticity. There are many studies reporting that IGF-I levels are low in delirium cases, and this low level is associated with the severity and duration of disease (Adamis et al. 2009). Mechanisms associated with the role of IGF-I, which has such metabolic effect, in the development of delirium are (Adamis and Meagher 2011):

*Neuroprotective IGF-I*: It may be effective in the pathogenesis of delirium due particularly to its cortical, hippocampal, and dopaminergic neuroprotective activity. IGF-I plays protective role for the neurons in the situations that lead to neurotoxicity such as hypoglycemia, hyperglycemia, β-amyloid toxicity, osmotic stress, deficiency of growth factors, low potassium and ceramide. Apoptosis is the mechanism which is most emphasized for cell death during neuronal injury. IGF-I prevents apoptosis by activating PI3K/Akt kinase and Ras/Raf/MEK/ERK pathways in the early phase and protein synthesis pathways (such as bcl-xL) in the late phase after neuronal injury. While decrease in IGF-I levels causes delirium by enhancing neuronal stress sensitivity, increased IGF-I levels may play an active role in the improvement of clinical.

*Impairment in somatotropic axis*: IGF-I plays an active role in GRH/somatostatin-growth hormone (GH)-IGF-I axis. GH has tropic effects on cognitive functions, mood, concentration, and general metabolism.

*Glucocorticoids-cytokines*: The facts that IGF-I is effective in the control of hypothalamo-pituitary-adrenal (HPA) axis and that increased glucocorticoids in delirium has decreasing effect on IGF-I expression are important for the development of delirium. Interaction between cytokines and IGF-I, oversensitivity of HPA axis in response to acute stress, and suppression of somatotropic axis may play a role in the development of delirium (Cerejeira et al. 2013).

## 2.4 Impairment in Sleep Pattern

Sleep is a process necessary for the regulation of physical and mental daily functions (Maldonado 2008). Biological clock and day light as well as melatonin are effective in the regulation of circadian rhythm of sleep. Melatonin is secreted from pineal gland under the control of suprachiasmatic nucleus in response to darkness. In a study, it was demonstrated that low melatonin levels were associated with in advanced age, delirium, postoperative period, and in the intensive care unit patients in whom sleep-alertness cycle is impaired (de Jonghe et al. 2010). Impairment in sleep regulation may cause memory problems, and this may be effective in the development of delirium in all inpatients especially in intensive care units. In the event of chronic partial sleeplessness defined as sleeping less than 4 h each night for consecutive 5 days, it was also demonstrated impairment in attention, judgment, reaction time, and recall functions of memory. Moreover, emotional imbalance such as irritability and fluctuation of mood due to the impaired interaction between amygdala and prefrontal cortex has been reported in the event of sleeplessness for more than 36 h. Based on these findings, inadequate sleep may cause both psychosis and delirium. Inadequate sleep not only causes delirium but also enhances severity and prolongs the duration of already existing delirium. It was determined that disturbance of sleep-alertness cycle and nighttime alertness in delirium resulted from irregular melatonin secretion (Misra and Ganzini 2003).

Interaction between immune system and sleep is also very important. Cytokine synthesis of immune system plays an active role in normal sleep cycle. Decrease in natural killer cell count, antibody levels after influenza vaccination, IL-2 production, and lymphokine-activated killer cell activity were determined in the situations of both acute and chronic sleeplessness. In addition, inadequate sleep can also influence endocrine and metabolic functions by altering cortisol secretion pattern and glucocorticoid feedback regulation (Spiegel et al. 1999; Ozturk et al. 1999). All of these explain the close physiological relationship between sleep and delirium.

## 2.5 Genetic

Although genetic-delirium relationship has been investigated in a very few studies and despite the data that genetic profile may increase the risk of delirium, the relationship between delirium and apolipoprotein E4 allele has been evaluated in the majority of studies, but no relation could have been demonstrated. The genetics of delirium tremens has been investigated more frequently and emphasis has been put on three different genes which play a role in dopamine transmission. However, no significant relationship has been found yet between these genes and delirium in elderly patients (Van Munster et al. 2009).

## 2.6 Drugs

Drugs, which are one of the main topics of geriatrics practice, are one of the most common causes of delirium. Different groups of drugs can cause delirium; however, sedative-hypnotics with documented psychoactive effect, narcotics, and anticholinergic drugs are the most frequently encountered ones. Particularly using more than five drugs enhances the risk of delirium in elderly patients. Since the prevention of development of disease is at least as important as treatment, drugs that facilitate development of delirium should be certainly known (Inouye 1998; Hubbard et al. 2013). It would be correct to say that the incidence of delirium in elderly patients will significantly decrease with discontinuation of psychoactive drugs in this population. The age-related changes in drug metabolism and elimination, as well as increase in the susceptibility against the drugs effective in the CNS, likely could be the cause of this (Lauretani et al. 2010). Other causes include:

- Polypharmacy
- Lack of information on drug-drug interaction in multiple drug usage
- Drug-disease interaction
- Age-related decrease in neurotransmitter production

Because many neurotransmitters, cytokines, and hormones take place in the pathogenesis of disease, it can be said that drugs that potentially influence these factors may play role in the development of delirium. In this topic, due to the plenty of the evidences that support cholinergic insufficiency, anticholinergic drugs should be taken account. In addition, the drugs that cause acetylcholine-dopamine imbalance in delirium should be kept in mind, too (Lauretani et al. 2010).

Digoxin unfavorably influences neuronal activity not only due to antimuscarinic effect but also by inhibiting membrane N-K-ATPase pump. Quinolone group antibiotics have mild dopaminergic effect as well as NMDA and GABA receptor antagonism. Morphine increases dopamine secretion and inhibits neuronal membrane N-K-ATPase pump. Histamine receptor blockers have both antimuscarinic effect and dopamine secretion. In addition, since alternative medicine is preferable for older people, hallucinogens such as mandrake, jimsonweed, and henbane among complementary medicines may also cause delirium (Alagiakrishnan and Wiens 2004).

It was reported that GABA transmission decreases and subsequently glutamate, NMDA, and dopaminergic and noradrenergic transmissions increase in delirium related to alcohol, sedative, or hypnotic withdrawn (Maldonado 2008).

In conclusion, all the etiological factors that play a role in the development of delirium unfavorably influence functional integration of cortical, prefrontal, and parietal networks, as well as subcortical structures such as basal ganglia, cerebellum, thalamic nuclei, and RAS. Furthermore, high cognitive processes such as attention, study memory, and administrative functions are impaired (Lauretani et al. 2010). However, pathogenesis of delirium has not been correctly explained by focusing only on a single mechanism (Watt et al. 2012; NICE 2010; Hovorka et al. 2012).

*Personal tendency*: Interaction between personal susceptibility and underlying reasons is important for risk factors of delirium considered as individual susceptibility. As defined in previous studies, while delirium can develop due to very simple reasons in high-risk cases as in older people, major causes may be enough to develop delirium in young, healthy, and low-risk cases (Inouye et al. 2014).

*Iatrogenic factors*: They are quite important in the development of delirium in elderly inpatients. Polypharmacy, anticholinergic drugs, and physical limitation at the time of hospitalization, monitoring, and impaired sleep routine are effective in the development of delirium (Inouye et al. 2014).

Although, multiple physiopathological mechanisms that take place in delirium have not been completely exposed yet, risk factors and facilitators could have been detected clearly. This is particularly important for the determination of preventive approaches.

## References

Adamis D, Meagher D (2011) Insulin-like growth factor i and the pathogenesis of delirium: a review of current evidence. J Aging Res 951403:1–11

Adamis D, Lunn M, Martin FC et al (2009) Cytokines and IGF-I in delirious and non-delirious acutely ill older medical inpatients. Age Ageing 38(3):326–332

Alagiakrishnan K, Wiens CA (2004) An approach to drug induced delirium in the elderly. Postgrad Med J 80:388–393

Ali MS, Harmer M, Vaughan R (2000) Serum S100 protein as a marker of cerebral damage during cardiac surgery. Br J Anaesth 85(2):287–298

Benbadis SR, Sila CA, Cristea RL (1994) Mental status changes and stroke. J Gen Intern Med 9:485

Brydon L, Harrison NA, Walker C, Steptoe A, Critchley HD (2008) Peripheral inflammation is associated with altered substantia nigra activity and psychomotor slowing in humans. Biol Psychiatry 63(11):1022–1029

Cerejeir J, Firmino H, Vaz-Serra A et al (2010) The neuroinflammatory hypothesis of delirium. Acta Neuropathol 119:737–754

Cerejeira J, Mukaetova-Ladinska EB (2011) A clinical update on delirium: from early recognition to effective management. Nurs Res Pract 875196:1–12

Cerejeira J, Batista P, Nogueira V et al (2011) Low preoperative plasma cholinesterase activity as a risk marker of postoperative delirium in elderly patients. Age Ageing 40:621–626

Cerejeira J, Batista P, Nogueira V et al (2013) The stress response to surgery and postoperative delirium: evidence of hypothalamic-pituitary-adrenal axis hyperresponsiveness and decreased suppression of the GH/IGF-1 axis. J Geriatr Psychiatry Neurol 26(3):185–194

Cole M, McCusker J, Dendukuri N, Han L (2003) The prognostic significance of subsyndromal delirium in elderly medical inpatients. J Am Geriatr Soc 51(6):754–760

Dimitrijevic OB, Stamatovic SM, Keep RF et al (2006) Effects of the chemokine CCL2 on blood-brain barrier permeability during ischemia-reperfusion injury. J Cereb Blood Flow Metab 26(6):797–810

Gao F, Harris DN, Sapsed-Byrne S (1999) Time course of neuron-specific enolase and S-100 protein release during and after coronary artery bypass grafting. Br J Anaesth 82(2):266–267

Hofer S, Bopp C, Hoerner C et al (2008) Injury of the blood brain barrier and up-regulation of ICAM-1 in polymicrobial sepsis. J Surg Res 146:276–281

Hovorka J, Mainerova B, Prasko J et al (2012) Delirium. Act Nerv Super Rediviva 54(4):180–191

Hshieh TT, Fong TG, Marcantonio ER, Inouye SK (2008) Cholinergic deficiency hypothesis in delirium: a synthesis of current evidence. J Gerontol A Biol Sci Med Sci 63(7):764–772

Hubbard RE, O'Mahony MS, Woodhouse KW (2013) Medication prescribing in frail older people. Eur J Clin Pharmacol 69:319–326

Inouye SK (1998) Delirium in hospitalized older patients: recognition and risk factors. J Geriatr Psychiatry Neurol 11(3):118–125

Inouye SK, Westendorp RGJ, Saczynski JS (2014) Delirium in elderly people. Lancet 383:911–922

Isik AT (2009) Approach to elderly patient with altered mental status. "Emergencies in Geriatrics and Geriatric Psychiatry". SomKitap, Istanbul, TURKEY, pp 23–44. ISBN:978-605-60355-1-7

Isik AT (2014) Delirium in the Elderly. İzmir Guven Kitap, Izmir, Turkey. ISBN:978-605-60355 de Jonghe A, Korevaar JC, van Munster BC et al (2010) Effectiveness of melatonin treatment on circadian rhythm disturbances in dementia. Are there implications for delirium? A systematic review. Rooij. Int J Geriatr Psychiatry 25:1201–1208

Krabbe KS, Reichenberg A, Yirmiya R, Smed A, Pedersen BK, Bruunsgaard H (2005) Low-dose endotoxemia and human neuropsychological functions. Brain Behav Immun 19(5):453–460

Krzyszton CP, Sparkman NL, Grant RW et al (2008) Exacerbated fatigue and motor deficits in interleukin-10-deficient mice after peripheral immune stimulation. Am J Physiol Regul Integr Comp Physiol 295(4):R1109–R1114

Lauretani F, Ceda GP, Maggio M et al (2010) Capturing side-effect of medication to identify persons at risk of delirium. Aging Clin Exp Res 22(5–6):456–458

Lee JW, Lee YK, Yuk DY et al (2008) Neuro-inflammation induced by lipopolysaccharide causes cognitive impairment through enhancement of beta-amyloid generation. J Neuroinflamm 5:37

Mac Lullich AMJ, Beaglehole A, Hall RJ, Meagher DJ (2009) Delirium and long-term cognitive impairment. Int Rev Psychiatry 21(1):30–42

Maldonado JR (2008) Pathoetiological model of delirium: comprehensive understanding of the neurobiology of delirium and an evidence-based approach to prevention and treatment. Crit Care Clin 24:789–856

Malek-Ahmadi P, Hilsabeck RC (2007) Neuropsychiatric complications of interferons: classification, neurochemical bases, and management. Ann Clin Psychiatry 19(2):113–123

Marchi N, Cavaglia M, Fazio V, Bhudia S, Hallene K, Janigro D (2004) Peripheral markers of blood-brain barrier damage. Clin Chim Acta 342(1–2):1

Martins S, Fernandes L (2012) Delirium in elderly people: a review. Front Neurol 3:101

Matto SK, Grover S, Gupta N (2010) Delirium in general practice. Indian J Med Res 131:387–398

McAfoose J, Baune BT (2009) Evidence for a cytokine model of cognitive function. Neurosci Biobehav Rev 33(3):355–366

McCaffrey G, Willis CL, Staatz WD et al (2009) Occludin oligomeric assemblies at tight junctions of the blood-brain barrier are altered by hypoxia and reoxygenation stress. J Neurochem 110(1):58–71

Misra S, Ganzini L (2003) Delirium, depression, and anxiety. Crit Care Clin 19(4):771–787

Mittal V, Muralee S, Williamson et al (2011) Delirium in the elderly: a comprehensive review. Am J Alzheimers Dis Other Demen 26(2) 97–109

Mullington J, Korth C, Hermann DM et al (2000) Dose-dependent effects of endotoxin on human sleep. Am J Physiol Regul Integr Comp Physiol 278(4):R947–R955

van Munster BC, Korevaar JC, Korse CM, Bonfrer JM, Zwinderman AH, de Rooij SE (2010) Serum S100B in elderly patients with and without delirium. Int J Geriatr Psychiatry 25(3): 234–239

National Institute for Clinical Excellence (NICE) (2010) Delirium: diagnosis, prevention and management, vol 3. NICE Clinical Guideline, London, pp 1–29

Nguyen DN, Spapen H, Su F et al (2006) Elevated serum levels of S-100beta protein and neuron-specific enolase are associated with brain injury in patients with severe sepsis and septic shock. Crit Care Med 34(7):1967–1974

Nishioku T, Dohgu S, Takata F et al (2009) Detachment of brain pericytes from the basal lamina is involved in disruption of the blood-brain barrier caused by lipopolysaccharide-induced sepsis in mice. Cell Mol Neurobiol 29(3):309–316

Noble F, Rubira E, Boulanouar M et al (2007) Acute systemic inflammation induces central mitochondrial damage and Mnesic deficit in adult Swiss mice. Neurosci Lett 424(2):106–110

O'Keeffe ST, Nı´ Chonchubhair A (1994) Postoperative delirium in the elderly. Br J Anaesth 73(5):673–687

Oztas B, Akgül S, Arslan FB (2004) Influence of surgical pain stress on the blood-brain barrier permeability in rats. Life Sci 74(16):1973–1979

Ozturk L, Pelin Z, Karadeniz D et al (1999) Effects of 48 hours sleep deprivation on human immune profile. Sleep Res Online 2(4):107–111

Qin L, Wu X, Block ML et al (2007) Systemic LPS causes chronic neuroinflammation and progressive neurodegeneration. Glia 55(5):453–462

Rachal Pugh C, Fleshner M, Watkins LR, Maier SF, Rudy JW (2001) The immune system and memory consolidation: a role for the cytokine IL-1beta. Neurosci Biobehav Rev 25(1):29–41

Reichenberg A, Yirmiya R, Schuld A et al (2001) Cytokine associated emotional and cognitive disturbances in humans. Arch Gen Psychiatry 58(5):445–452

Richwine AF, Sparkman NL, Dilger RN, Buchanan JB, Johnson RW (2009) Cognitive deficits in interleukin-10-deficient mice after peripheral injection of lipopolysaccharide. Brain Behav Immun 23(6):794–802

Semmler A, Okulla T, Sastre M, Dumitrescu-Ozimek L, Heneka M (2005) Systemic inflammation induces apoptosis with variable vulnerability of different brain regions. J Chem Neuroanat 30:144–157

Sharshar T, Gray F, Lorin de la Grandmaison G et al (2003) Apoptosis of neurons in cardiovascular autonomic centres triggered by inducible nitric oxide synthase after death from septic shock. Lancet 362(9398):1799–1805

Sharshar T, Carlier R, Bernard F et al (2007) Brain lesions in septic shock: a magnetic resonance imaging study. Intensive Care Med 33(5):798–806

Siami S, Annane D, Sharshar T (2008) The encephalopathy in sepsis. Crit Care Clin 24(1):67–82

Sparkman NL, Buchanan JB, Heyen JR, Chen J, Beverly JL, Johnson RW (2006) Interleukin-6 facilitates lipopolysaccharide-induced disruption in working memory and expression of other proinflammatory cytokines in hippocampal neuronal cell layers. J Neurosci 26(42):10709–10716

Spiegel K, Leproult R, Van Cauter E (1999) Impact of sleep debt on metabolic and endocrine function. Lancet 354(9188):1435–1439

Tanaka S, Ide M, Shibutani T et al (2006) Lipopolysaccharide-induced microglial activation induces learning and memory deficits without neuronal cell death in rats. J Neurosci Res 83(4):557–566

Terry AV, Buccafusco JJ (2003) The cholinergic hypothesis of age and Alzheimer's disease-related cognitive deficits: recent challenges and their implications for novel drug development. J Pharmacol Exp Ther 306:821–827

Tizard I (2008) Sickness behavior, its mechanisms, significance. Anim Health Res Rev 9(1):87–99

Tracey KJ (2009) Reflex control of immunity. Nat Rev Immunol 9(6):418–428

Trzepacz PT (1994) The neuropathogenesis of delirium: a need to focus our research. Psychosomatics 35:374

Uchikado H, Akiyama H, Kondo H et al (2004) Activation of vascular endothelial cells and perivascular cells by systemic inflammation-an immunohistochemical study of postmortem human brain tissues. Acta Neuropathol 107(4):341–351

Van Der Mast RC (1998) Pathophysiology of delirium. J Geriat Psychiatr Neurol 11:138–145

Van Munster BC, de Rooij SE, Korevaar JC (2009) The role of genetics in delirium in the elderly patient. Dement Geriatr Cogn Disord 28(3):187–195

Watt DF, Koziol K, Budding D (2012) Delirium and confusional states. In: Noggleand CA, Dean RS (eds) Disorders in neuropsychiatry. Springer, New York

Weinberger DR (1993) A connectionist approach to the prefrontal cortex. J Neuropsychiatry Clin Neurosci 5(3):241–253

White S (2002) The neuropathogenesis of delirium. Rev Clin Gerontol 12:62–67

# Delirium: Clinical Features, Diagnosis and Differential Diagnosis

# 3

Ismet Kirpinar

Delirium is an acute brain dysfunction which develops over a short period of time and may result from several different aetiologies. It is characterized by disturbance in various cognitive functions primarily of attention and awareness. It can develop easily in the elderly who are already vulnerable with several predisposing and precipitating factors. Delirium is a common, serious and often fatal disorder that affects as many as 50% of people older than 65 years who are admitted to the hospital (Inouye et al. 2014). The significance of delirium is not limited to its high prevalence; at the same time, it has marked negative effects on various parameters such as medical morbidity, duration of hospital stay and outcome after discharge (Cole and Primeau 1993; Fong et al. 2009). Delirium is an alarming sign that underlying medical condition is serious to an extent of increasing mortality and morbidity rates. It may not be recognized in the elderly patient and might be misinterpreted as dementia, depression or a natural course of ageing.

## 3.1 Clinical Features

Delirium is defined as a reversible and temporary impairment of brain function. It is a syndrome, not a disease, and it has many causes, all of which result in a similar pattern of signs and symptoms. The type and severity of signs vary depending on the patient and the aetiology. However, common signs and symptoms which make the core syndrome are similar. The essential feature of delirium is a disturbance of attention or awareness that is accompanied by a change in baseline cognition that cannot be better explained by a preexisting or evolving neurocognitive disorder (American Psychiatric Association 2013).

I. Kirpinar, M.D.
Department of Psychiatry, Faculty of Medicine, Bezmialem Vakif University, Vatan Cad., İstanbul, Turkey
e-mail: ikirpinar@yahoo.com



A.T. Isik, G.T. Grossberg (eds.), *Delirium in Elderly Patients*,
https://doi.org/10.1007/978-3-319-65239-9_3

### 3.1.1 Onset of Symptoms

One of the most characteristic features of delirium is rapid development of its symptoms. The symptoms usually emerge within hours or days. The onset sometimes may be abrupt. The relatives or carers might state that the patient was well until a short while ago and that it all changed suddenly. Relatives and care staff may describe features such as an acute change or decline in function, disturbed sleep/wake cycle or sleeplessness, rapid memory decline, 'confusion' or a rapid change in personality or behaviour. This type of onset helps differentiate delirium from other neurocognitive disorders mainly dementia.

### 3.1.2 Prodromal Phase

In some patients there could be prodromal changes for 1–3 days before the onset of florid symptoms. Patients might appear irritable, perplexed and restless. In cases where the onset is more gradual, there could be mild and temporary symptoms such as anxiety, decreased concentration, fatigue and sleep problems (Krahne et al. 2006). In some patients certain cognitive impairments like mild confusion or difficulty in remembering and hypersensitivity to light and sound and changes in perception can be noticeable. The most commonly seen sign is sleep disturbance like daytime sleepiness. Prodromal signs can recede after a short while or can develop into a marked delirium. The presence of prodromal signs should be taken into consideration when elderly patients are treated both in the inpatient and outpatient settings and during their first presentation for assessment. The interventions for diagnosis and treatment towards general medical conditions could prevent development of a likely delirium syndrome.

### 3.1.3 Fluctuating Course

Fluctuations and changes in severity and type of symptoms are one of the most typical features of delirium. Fluctuation in clinical manifestation with worsening in attention, awareness and other realms of cognitive function interspersed with periods of lucid intervals during the course of the day is a diagnostic feature of delirium. A somnolent patient can become fully alert and later on within minutes can get worse with agitation. This feature undoubtedly is one of the most important reasons why diagnosis can be overlooked in patients who are not assessed frequently. These fluctuations in symptoms and intermittent worsening are unpredictable and irregular; however, there is often some improvement during the daytime and worsening at night.

### 3.1.4 Signs and Symptoms

There are various signs and symptoms of delirium. Although most of these can be seen during the course of normal ageing or dementia, some are typically seen in delirium. When Gottlieb et al. (1991) compared two groups of hospitalized elderly patients with and without delirium by using DSM-III criteria, clouding of consciousness, disorientation, memory impairment, fluctuation and acute onset were present in 100% of patients with delirium, while the same symptoms were present in 5%, 34%, 64%, 9% and 12%, respectively, of patients without delirium. Similarly, perceptual disturbances, incoherent speech, sleep disorder and psychomotor changes occurred in 75%, 76%, 96% and 93%, respectively, of delirious patients and 3%, 6%, 65% and 40%, respectively, of non-delirious patients. The review studies of delirium cases done in the 1990s showed the most common signs of delirium as follows: clouding of consciousness (65–100%), disorganized thinking (95%) and short-term memory and recall difficulties (62–90%) (Meagher and Trzepacz 1998; Trzepacz 1999).

In delirium, depending on the personal vulnerability, cognitive capacity and the type and severity of underlying pathology, all or some of the symptoms described below can be seen. For a diagnosis of delirium, those symptoms or signs may not be evident all the time as they will fluctuate, but they must be of recent onset.

- Disturbances in consciousness: Consciousness is described as being aware of internal and external stimuli. For consciousness, a normal level of arousal is required but not sufficient. It also requires to be able to give appropriate responses to stimuli. Disturbance in consciousness is a cardinal feature of delirium, but it is difficult to describe and examine it. In reality, consciousness shows a continuum from hyperalertness/hyperarousal to coma. For a diagnosis of delirium, the Diagnostic and Statistical Manual of Mental Disorders, 5th edition (DSM-V), requires that impairment in attention and other cognitive functions do not occur in the context of a severely reduced level of arousal, such as coma (American Psychiatric Association 2013). However, low-level arousal states with minimal responses should be considered in the context of delirium. In some patients disturbances in consciousness can manifest itself as hyperalertness/hyperarousal or with lethargy and reduced arousal in others. In delirium patients may not be woken up fully and can fall asleep easily, or there could be increased attention with excessive alertness and startle reaction. Some patients might fluctuate between the two extremes during the course of the day.
- Reduced ability to direct, focus, sustain and shift attention: Attention is a process of direction and focus of perception towards selected stimuli. The maintenance of this process for certain activities and attending to various stimuli simultaneously is described as the content of attention. Impairment in attention is the most characteristic feature of delirium. This can be assessed by observing the ability of patient following the instruction during the medical examination/interview. Patients have difficulty focusing on the stimulus, and the question/stimulus needs to be repeated in order to get a response. The ability of attention can be objectively assessed by some bedside tests.
- Disorientation: Impairment in orientation is the most common sign of delirium. Besides being a common sign, it plays a main role for recognizing delirium. People can be easily assessed by asking about the place and time they are in

which is quite useful for a diagnosis of delirium. It is particularly important to do regular assessments on the elderly vulnerable patients for early recognition and treatment. Disorientation may occur in time (not knowing what time of day, day of week, month, season or year), place (not knowing where one is) or person (not knowing who one is). The earliest and most common impairment is seen in temporal orientation. Disorientation to person is very rare and indicates the seriousness of the condition.

- Disorganized thinking and speech: In most delirious elderly patients, the clarity, consistency and the speed of speech get impaired. There could be inconsistent flow of thoughts with loosening of associations between the words, sentences and topics. This is known as disorganized thinking which is observed as a difficulty to understand and inconsistent speech. Other speech and language disturbances such as dysarthria, dysnomia, dysgraphia and even aphasia may occur in delirium.
- Memory disturbances: Short-term memory problems and difficulties with remembering are common problems in delirium. However, these impairments are temporary and unlike in dementia are not a result of a neurodegenerative process and are due to fluctuations in consciousness and disturbance in attention. There is impairment in registration, recall and recognition. It impacts short-term memory more than long-term memory (American Psychiatric Association 2013). There could be no problem with easy short-term memory tasks such as repeating a word or answering simple questions. However, there are usually problems with relatively difficult tasks throughout the delirium such as repeating a telephone number. Registration of newly learned knowledge in the long-term memory requires high-level concentration which is often impaired in delirium. Recalling old memories does not require concentration which is generally not effected in delirium. However, in cases where the underlying pathology causes severe brain damage, long-term memory can also get disturbed as a result, not because of delirium itself.
- Sleep-wake disturbances: Sleep-wake cycle disturbances are very common in delirium and have been proposed as a core criterion for the diagnosis. Due to impairment of circadian sleep cycle, there are sleep-wake rhythm disturbances in most patients with excessive sleepiness during the daytime and increased alertness at night. Decreased or broken sleep at night could be the first sign of delirium in many patients. Patients wake up with vivid dreams and nightmares. They can confuse dreams with real life due to sleepless nights and excessive sleepiness during the day.
- Perceptual disturbances: Hallucinations, misperceptions, illusions and delusions are reported to occur in at least 40% of cases of delirium (Cole et al. 2002). Perceptual disturbances are usually visual but may occur in other modalities. They are mostly illusions. Patients might, for example, misperceive the blood pressure device that a nurse is using as a weapon or a water pipe in the room as snake or folds in bed as various animals. Hallucinations are perceptions without external stimuli. Hallucinations are usually visual, ranging from dreamlike experiences to terrifying visions. They are particularly common in patients with

delirium due to multiple aetiologies and receiving more active medical treatment (Webster and Holroyd 2000). They are experienced mostly at night, when it is dark and when the patient is alone. When there's no one around, they might see a group of people around the bed, dangerous animals or strange figures. There could be interesting hallucinations like macropsia (a disorder of visual perception in which objects appear larger than their actual size) or micropsia (seeing tiny human or animal figures). Less frequently auditory hallucinations or those involving taste and smell may occur. There could be very disturbing tactile hallucinations particularly in deliriums secondary to alcohol/substance withdrawal.

- Emotional disturbances: Emotional changes can last long which can be reported as personality change by others or can be intermittent changes with lability. There is no mood or affect changes specific to delirium. However, there are often disturbances in the form of anxiety, anger, apathy, depression, euphoria or irritability.
- Thought content: There are often persecutory delusions in thought content (they will kill me; they will slaughter me). Misperceptions (a nurse preparing a medicine can be perceived as if he/she is trying to poison the patient) can lead to these thoughts. Delusions are short-lived and temporary and are not considered as fixed delusions.
- Altered psychomotor activity: This is one of the most important signs of delirium making the monitoring of the patients difficult. It varies according to the type of delirium which will be discussed below. Patients with hyperactive delirium show increased alertness and hypervigilance. They can be agitated, disruptive and aggressive. On the other hand, hypoactive ones are sleepy with marked motionlessness and retardation.
- Other features: Higher integrative functions are affected; the result is a reduced ability to plan and solve problems or disrupted sequencing or praxis of actions (e.g. rising from a bed or walking which can lead to injury or falls). Disturbances can also occur in visuospatial abilities and in writing. It is important to note that the sensory features tend to be less common in elderly than in younger patients. Somatic features such as urinary incontinence, gait impairment, tremor and language disorders (including receptive and expressive dysphasia) tend to be more common in older people with delirium (Lipowski 1980).

## 3.2 Clinical Subtypes

Based on the levels of arousal and psychomotor functions, three types of delirium are described (Lipowski 1983; Meagher et al. 1996). It has been suggested that each delirium subtype can result from different pathophysiological mechanisms and that each might carry a different prognosis (Fong et al. 2009).

*Hyperactive delirium* which is marked by increased psychomotor activity occurs in 15–46% of delirium patients (Meagher et al. 1996; Liptzin and Levkoff 1992; Marcantonio et al. 2002; Camus et al. 2000; Margiotta et al. 2006). There is hyperarousal with increased sensitivity to immediate surroundings to the point where patients can be verbally and physically aggressive. Patients present with repetitive behaviours such as plucking at sheets, picking or pulling the bed linens, rubbing his/her genitals, attempting to get out of bed and wandering or perceptual disturbances such as illusions or hallucinations. Patients with hyperactive delirium have shorter hospital stay comparing to other subtypes, and they are accepted to have better prognosis. This variant of delirium is most commonly recognized and tends to be readily apparent even to the casual observer. It is often associated with the adverse effects of anticholinergic drugs, drug intoxication and withdrawal states. Characteristically, patients may exhibit agitation, psychosis and mood lability, may refuse to cooperate with medical care, may demonstrate disruptive behaviours (such as shouting or resisting) and may sustain injuries from falling, combativeness or pulling out catheters and intravascular lines (Rummans et al. 1995; Rudberg et al. 1997).

*Hypoactive delirium* which occurs in 19–71% of patients is typically unrecognized or misattributed to dementia or depression (Spronk et al. 2009; Meagher et al. 1996; O'Keeffe and Lavan 1999; Liptzin and Levkoff 1992; Marcantonio et al. 2002). Some researchers are of the opinion that due to the restriction of diagnostic criteria in DSM, actual higher rates are not detected (Treloar and Macdonald 1997). Hypoactive type is also described as somnolent type which is marked by psychomotor slowing and withdrawal and may be misidentified as depression (Ross et al. 1991). Patients appear quiet, withdrawn and lethargic and present with clouding of consciousness with reduced mobility/movement. They often have daytime sleepiness. Spontaneous movements and speech are slowed down a lot. Therefore communication can be provided with difficulty. They may need to be reminded several times to respond to the questions. These patients are confused and look tired. This is the most common type of delirium seen in the elderly patients. However, they can be easily overlooked because of being calm and sleepy, not displaying any aggression towards themselves or others and having no bizarre behaviours. It is known that hypoactive delirium is caused by severe, acute underlying pathologies such as infections, hypoxia, hypothermia, hyperglycaemia, hepatic and renal failures and thyroid diseases (O'Keeffe and Lavan 1999; Trzepacz 1994; Justic 2000). Delirium in the elderly is usually caused by these conditions; therefore, hypoactive type is thought be more often in this patient group.

*Mixed forms*: Mixed forms may occur in 43–56% of patients (O'Keeffe and Lavan 1999; Liptzin and Levkoff 1992). Patients with mixed delirium demonstrate both hyperactive and hypoactive features. This presentation is marked by obvious fluctuations in activity level, cognitive disturbance, level of consciousness and organization of thinking. There is usually sedation, sleepiness and no movement during the daytime while agitation, increased activity and disruptive behaviour at night.

Certain types of delirium may frequently occur in patients with particular disease states; however, they are neither exclusive nor diagnostic of specific underlying medical conditions. Similarly, the manifestation of delirium cannot be fully predicted by the presence of a particular aetiological toxin or illness. Because of the multiple aetiological factors, the fluctuating course and the individual medical comorbidities, many patients who experience delirium have a mixture of both hypoactive and hyperactive variants. Some studies suggest that such patients present the greatest risk of substantial morbidity and mortality (Stagno et al. 2004).

In an observational study done on 225 prospective admissions to the geriatric unit of a training hospital, it was founded out that from 94 admissions with delirium, 20 (21%) had a hyperactive delirium, 27 (29%) had a hypoactive delirium, 40 (43%) had a mixed hypoactive-hyperactive psychomotor pattern and 7 (7%) had no psychomotor disturbances. Patients with hypoactive delirium were sicker on admission, had the longest hospital stay and were most likely to develop pressure sores. Patients with hyperactive delirium were most likely to have a fall in the hospital. There were no differences in aetiological factors between the groups (O'Keeffe and Lavan 1999).

## 3.3 Diagnosis

The diagnosis of delirium is primarily clinical and is based on careful bedside observation of key features. There is no specific test. One should always suspect delirium when elderly patients particularly those with dementia present with acute or subacute disturbances in behaviour, cognition or functioning. There is a need for full physical examination with detailed history including mental state examination in these cases. The history should confirm that an acute change in baseline cognitive function has occurred. It is important to ascertain the time course of the mental status changes, as well as any history of intercurrent illnesses, medication usage (including any changes in medication and use of over-the-counter and herbal products), alcohol withdrawal and changes in the environment. Because patients with delirium are often confused and cannot give a proper history, the information obtained from family, carers and nurses is important. It is important to check nursing notes particularly for night-time disorientation, abnormal behaviour and perceptual disturbances.

### 3.3.1 Diagnostic Difficulties

Delirium is often unrecognized by the patients' physicians and nurses, in part because of its fluctuating nature, its overlap with dementia, lack of formal cognitive assessment and underappreciation of its clinical consequences (Saxena and Lawley 2009). The bedside mental status examinations and interviews show dramatic fluctuations. Therefore, cognitive assessments which will be performed at regular intervals in an elderly patient are too helpful to determine the developing delirium. It might not be likely to do standard cognitive tests particularly on patients at the surgical and intensive care units as they are intubated and cannot respond verbally to questions.

Hypoactive patients which comprise the majority of the delirium cases can be overlooked due to "quite" symptoms. It also makes measuring the changes from baseline difficult when there is not sufficient information on premorbid personality and functioning of the elderly patients. Cognitive/mental problems in the elderly patients with medical conditions are usually considered as reasonable or expected by relatives and hospital staff which can prevent to focus enough on delirium symptoms. Problems with the system or clinics such as ward transfers due to multiple medical problems and shift changes can also make the diagnosis difficult. Studies suggest that between a third and two thirds of delirium goes unrecognized (Siddiqi et al. 2006). In a study, it was shown that only 31% of the patients could be diagnosed with delirium. In the same study, it was determined that delirium diagnosis could not be made especially in the patients over 80 years with hypoactive delirium, visual problems and dementia diagnosis (Inouye et al. 2001). Another study measured nursing identification of delirium using standardized case vignettes, only 21% of nurses were able to correctly identify the hypoactive form of delirium superimposed on dementia (DSD) and 41% correctly identified hypoactive delirium alone in the case vignettes (Fick et al. 2007).

### 3.3.2 Diagnostic Criteria

The essential feature of delirium is a disturbance of consciousness and attention that is accompanied by a change in baseline cognition that cannot be better explained by another neurocognitive disorder. The appearance of symptoms within a short period of time like hours or days and the fluctuation of symptoms during the course of the day are the diagnostic features related to the course of delirium. In addition to these criteria, there is evidence from the history, physical examination or laboratory findings that the disturbance is a physiological consequence of a general medical condition.

A formal diagnosis can be made by using the DSM-V or International Classification of Diseases 10 (ICD-10) criteria (American Psychiatric Association 2013; World Health Organization 1992). Diagnosis of delirium according to the DSM-V requires disturbance of attention and awareness; change in cognition (including memory deficit, disorientation or language disturbance); development over a short period of time, usually hours to a few days; fluctuations during the course of the day; and evidences from the history, physical examination or laboratory findings that the disturbance is a physiological consequence of an underlying medical condition, substance intoxication or withdrawal, use of a medication or a toxin exposure or a combination of these factors (Table 3.1).

DSM-V recognizes seven diagnostic categories:

1. Substance intoxication delirium
2. Substance withdrawal delirium
3. Medication-induced delirium
4. Delirium due to another medical condition
5. Delirium due to multiple aetiologies
6. Other specified delirium
7. Unspecified delirium

**Table 3.1** DSM-V diagnostic criteria for delirium

| | |
|---|---|
| A. | A disturbance in attention (i.e. reduced ability to direct, focus, sustain and shift attention) and awareness (reduced orientation to the environment) |
| B. | The disturbance develops over a short period of time (usually hours to a few days), represents a change from baseline attention and awareness and tends to fluctuate in severity during the course of a day |
| C. | An additional disturbance in cognition (e.g. memory deficit, disorientation, language, visuospatial ability or perception) |
| D. | The disturbances in Criteria A and C are not better explained by another preexisting, established or evolving neurocognitive disorder and do not occur in the context of a severely reduced level of arousal, such as coma |
| E. | There is evidence from the history, physical examination or laboratory findings that the disturbance is a direct physiological consequence of another medical condition, substance intoxication or withdrawal (i.e. due to a drug of abuse or to a medication) or exposure to a toxin or is due to multiple aetiologies |
| *Specify* if: | |
| Acute: Lasting a few hours or days | |
| Persistent: Lasting weeks or months | |
| *Specify* if: | |
| Hyperactive: The individual has a hyperactive level of psychomotor activity that may be accompanied by mood lability, agitation and/or refusal to cooperate with medical care | |
| Hypoactive: The individual has a hypoactive level of psychomotor activity that may be accompanied by sluggishness and lethargy that approaches stupor | |
| Mixed level of activity: The individual has a normal level of psychomotor activity even though attention and awareness are disturbed. Also includes individuals whose activity level rapidly fluctuates | |

Diagnostic criteria for delirium according to ICD-10 are shown in Table 3.2. The ICD-10 definition appears to be much narrower than DSM-IV. It has separate requirements for cognitive disturbance (which must be evidenced by impairment in immediate recall and recent memory with intact long-term memory and disorientation to time, place or person), one of four types of psychomotor disturbance and one of three specified manifestations of disturbance of the sleep-wake cycle.

### 3.3.3 Examination

Delirium remains a clinical diagnosis made on the basis of a detailed history, behavioural observation and cognitive assessment. A careful and complete physical examination including a mental status examination is necessary for the diagnosis. Establishing previous functional and cognitive status and recent events such as falls or medication changes is essential. For a proper diagnosis, it is necessary to do periodic assessment of diagnostic criteria and have information about baseline mental status of the patient. During the assessment, elderly patients should be provided with sensory aids such as spectacles or hearing aids.

It is a clear necessity to take history from a family member or carer in elderly patients who has medical problems. The history should confirm that an acute change in

**Table 3.2** ICD-10 diagnostic criteria for delirium

| |
|---|
| For a definite diagnosis, symptoms, mild or severe, should be present *in each one* of the following areas: |
| (a) Impairment of consciousness and attention (on a continuum from clouding to coma, reduced ability to direct, focus, sustain and shift attention) |
| (b) Global disturbance of cognition (perceptual distortions, illusions and hallucinations—most often visual; impairment of abstract thinking and comprehension, with or without transient delusions but typically with some degree of incoherence; impairment of immediate recall and of recent memory but with relatively intact remote memory; disorientation for time as well as, in more severe cases, for place and person) |
| (c) Psychomotor disturbances (hypo- or hyperactivity and unpredictable shifts from one to the other, increased reaction time, increased or decreased flow of speech, enhanced startle reaction) |
| (d) Disturbance of the sleep-wake cycle (insomnia or, in severe cases, total sleep loss or reversal of the sleep-wake cycle, daytime drowsiness, nocturnal worsening of symptoms, disturbing dreams or nightmares, which may continue as hallucinations after awakening) |
| (e) Emotional disturbances, e.g. depression, anxiety or fear, irritability, euphoria, apathy or wondering perplexity |
| The onset is usually rapid, the course diurnally fluctuating and the total duration of the condition less than 6 months. The above clinical picture is so characteristic that a fairly confident diagnosis of delirium can be made even if the underlying cause is not clearly established. In addition to a history of an underlying physical or brain disease, evidence of cerebral dysfunction (e.g. an abnormal electroencephalogram, usually but not invariably showing a slowing of the background activity) may be required if the diagnosis is in doubt |

baseline cognitive function has occurred. It is important to ascertain the time course of the mental status changes, as well as any history of intercurrent illnesses, medication usage (including any changes in medication and use of over-the-counter and herbal products), alcohol withdrawal and changes in the environment (Fong et al. 2009).

The main mental status change in delirious patients is cognitive impairment, and the most important risky group for delirium is hospitalized older people. The guidelines recommend that all clinical encounters with sick older people should routinely include assessment of cognition (Young and Inouye 2007; Michauda et al. 2007).

The key problem is fluctuations in consciousness. In order to assess consciousness level, patients can be given verbal, auditory or motor stimuli, and then they are assessed for their comprehension or responses. The Glasgow Coma Scale may be used to quantify level of consciousness (Teasdale and Jennett 1974; Teasdale 2014).

Attentional process can be evaluated by observing patient's ability to follow instructions and medical interventions. There are short bedside tests to assess attention. Digit Span and Continuous Performance tests are among the most commonly used ones. Digit span task involves asking the patient to say out loud a string of 4–6 digits after the assessor (Blackburn and Benton 1957). In continuous performance test, the patient is asked to put his hand up every time he hears letter X or A among a string of letters read out with 1 s interval during 30 s (Cornblatt et al. 1988). Assessment of orientation is easy and has an important role in diagnosis. It can be assessed by asking questions related to time, place and persons.

Bedside mental state examinations and interviews show dramatic fluctuations. Hence, this assessment should be carried out frequently in patients with delirium or at risk of developing one. Older patients should be aroused during rounds and evaluated daily for the hypoactive form of delirium, which is often overlooked.

### 3.3.4 Screening Instruments

In addition to a standard clinical interview, several screening tools and scales have been developed to identify patients with delirium. Simple cognitive tests for inpatients such as the Mini-Mental State Examination (MMSE), Standardized MMSE (SMMSE) and Clock Drawing Test (CDT) are not specific to delirium but still useful for screening and monitoring as they demonstrate cognitive dysfunction. It is recommended to perform these tests daily for early diagnosis in patients at risk (O'Keeffe et al. 2005). Mini-Cog, despite its limitations for sensitivity and predictive validity, is another test used to screen for cognitive impairment (Ismail et al. 2010).

There are several tools developed and validated to screen for delirium. It can help not to miss delirium in those who cannot talk such as patients at intensive care unit. The Confusion Assessment Method (CAM) is the most widely studied research tool in delirium and is perhaps the best tool for screening delirium (Inouye et al. 1990; Saxena and Lawley 2009). The CAM has four items based on the DSM-III-R criteria, which are determined by the patient, nurse and family interview. These features are as follows: (1) an acute onset of mental status changes or a fluctuating course, (2) inattention, (3) disorganized thinking and (4) an altered level of consciousness. The patient is diagnosed as delirious (i.e. CAM positive) if he or she has both features 1 and 2 and either feature 3 or 4. The CAM algorithm has a sensitivity of 94–100% and a specificity of 90–95%. It has a high inter-rater reliability when administered by trained interviewers. Most of US and UK guidelines recommend the CAM for routine use (Young and Inouye 2007).

Other frequently used tools are the Confusion Assessment Tool for Intensive Care Unit (CAM-ICU) (Ely et al. 2001), Intensive Care Delirium Screening Checklist (ICDSC) (Bergeron et al. 2001), Nursing Delirium Screening Scale (Nu-DESC) (Gaudreau et al. 2005) and NEECHAM Confusion Scale (Neelon et al. 1996). Informant Assessment of Geriatric Delirium Scale (I-AGeD) was developed to identify older people with delirium (Rhodius-Meester et al. 2013). Delirium Detection Score (DDS) is a useful scale to assess the degree of delirium and guide treatment, and the tool may also serve as a diagnostic scale (Otter et al. 2005). Delirium Rating Scale and Delirium Rating Scale-Revised-98 are the most commonly used tools to measure the severity of symptoms of delirium (Trzepacz et al. 2001).

It is extremely important to do a brief bedside neurological examination for a quick diagnosis in delirium like in all organic mental disorders. If there is suspicion of delirium, pupillary and fundoscopic examination should be carried out as well as checking for neck stiff ness. Patients with delirium can also demonstrate nonspecific focal findings, such as asterixis or tremor on neurological examination, although the presence of any new neurological deficit, particularly with accompanying focal neurological signs, should raise suspicion of an acute cerebrovascular event or subdural hematoma. In many elderly patients and in individuals with cognitive impairment, delirium could be the initial manifestation of a new serious disease (Fong et al. 2009). In speech, dysphasia (anomia) usually presents as systematic misnaming. Most of the time there is misnaming reflecting people's previous experiences. A carpenter patient, for example, can call the stethoscope pliers.

A full physical examination should be carried on every patient who presents with changes in mental state. Once a diagnosis of delirium has been established, the potential cause—in particular, any life-threatening contributors—must be determined. All preadmission and current medications should be reviewed. A medical history must be meticulously obtained to detect some medical emergencies. An examination of temperature, pulse rate, blood pressure and respiration must definitely be performed. Delirium should be considered to be a medical emergency until proven otherwise; mortality rates for patients admitted to hospital with delirium can range from 10 to 26% (McCusker et al. 2002). Basic medical care, including airway protection, assessment of vital signs and laboratory tests to exclude treatable conditions such as infections, should be administered (Fong et al. 2009).

In cases where it proves difficult to do all the examinations and assessments required due to agitation or restlessness, assessing vital signs is an easy way of obtaining valuable information. Particularly general appearance, vital signs, hydration status and signs of physical trauma should be meticulously assessed. Enlargement of thyroid, hear murmurs and cardiac arrhythmias should be looked for. Chest auscultation, abdominal examination for a possible liver or spleen enlargement and examination of the skin for jaundice or rash would very helpful. General appearance would point to some clues about substance or alcohol use. High fever, pupillary dilation or constriction and changes in respiratory rate, pulse rate and blood pressure can be diagnostic for certain medical conditions.

### 3.3.5 Laboratory Investigations

Laboratory tests for full blood count (helpful in infection and anaemia), electrolytes (high or low values) and glucose (hypoglycaemia, ketoacidosis); renal and liver function tests (renal and liver failure); thyroid function tests (hypothyroidism); urine sample (urinary tract infections); screening for substances in the urine (toxicological causes), thiamine and vit B12 levels (vitamin deficiencies); tests for bacteriologic and viral aetiologies (for infections) and sedimentation; screening for substance use including alcohol level; and tests for HIV and other infections if needed should be carried out. Neuroimaging is performed in selected patients to exclude a focal structural abnormality, such as an acute stroke, that might mimic delirium in its presentation (Fong et al. 2009).

## 3.4 Differential Diagnosis

Delirium can be confused with several psychiatric disorders due to various cognitive, behavioural and psychological symptoms. Variability of symptoms and the clinical picture of hypoactive and hyperactive types can make the diagnosis difficult in the majority of cases. Because of its primary presentation with cognitive symptoms in the older people, delirium mainly gets confused with other neurocognitive disorders especially dementia. However, it might still be difficult to distinguish it from other psychiatric disorders. Differential diagnosis is mostly based on the history, cognitive deterioration and the presence of underlying medical condition.

### 3.4.1 Distinguishing Delirium and Dementia (Major Neurocognitive Disorder)

"Dementia" describes a chronic and usually irreversible decline in cognitive and psychosocial functions. It usually results from an identifiable degenerative brain disease (e.g. Alzheimer's disease). Distinguishing delirium from dementia (which is subsumed under the newly named entity major neurocognitive disorder in DSM-V) is a common clinical dilemma. In order to make diagnosis of delirium or major neurocognitive disorder, DSM-V requires the exclusion of other diagnosis. "The cognitive deficits do not occur exclusively in the context of a delirium" for major neurocognitive disorder and "The disturbances are not better explained by another pre-existing, established, or evolving neurocognitive disorder" for delirium (American Psychiatric Association 2013). However, there is a strong interrelationship between delirium and dementia, both pathophysiological and clinical (Fick et al. 2002). First, delirium and dementia share the same clinical and psychological features to a great degree. Both are the most important causes of cognitive impairment and can mask each other. Second, dementia is the most important risk factor for delirium in the older patients (Margiotta et al. 2006; Pisani et al. 2007). Patients with dementia have already a fragile brain which is a high-risk factor delirium. The underlying vulnerability of the brain in patients with dementia may predispose them to the development of delirium as a result of insults related to acute medical illnesses, medications or environmental perturbations (Inouye 2006). Thus, delirium episodes can superimpose on a preexisting dementia, such as that due to Alzheimer's disease. Delirium superimposed on dementia (DSD) is increasingly problematic as the population ages. The prevalence of DSD ranges from 18 to 89% in hospitalized and community-dwelling older adults (Fick et al. 2002; Fong et al. 2009). Additionally, a co-existing major cognitive disorder can make the case of delirium more complicated. Finally, delirium can signal underlying vulnerability of the brain, with decreased cognitive reserve and increased risk for development of dementia in the future. Although it is not likely that the delirium itself causes the pathologic changes of dementia, severe precipitating factors such as prolonged hypoglycaemia or hypoxaemia can lead to permanent neuronal damage and dementia. Delirium might also mediate the effect of many factors, such as general surgery, anaesthesia, critical illness, acute respiratory distress syndrome, prolonged intubation or sepsis, on long-term cognitive outcomes. There is no question that delirium contributes to worsening functional status, loss of independence and poorer outcomes among patients with dementia (Inouye 2006).

Because of all the listed factors above, it is a complex task to distinguish delirium and dementia in older people. The clinician must determine whether the individual has delirium; a delirium superimposed on a preexisting NCD, such as that due to Alzheimer's disease; or an NCD without delirium. But the traditional distinction between delirium and dementia according to acuteness of onset and temporal course is particularly difficult in those elderly individuals who had a prior NCD that may not have been recognized or who develop persistent cognitive impairment following an episode of delirium. Clinical features may be useful in distinguishing delirium from Alzheimer or Lewy body dementia. An impaired consciousness with fluctuating levels is one of the most helpful symptoms in the diagnosis of delirium. Although disorientation is substantially typical for delirium, it can be hard to examine the patients with memory impairment or amnesia. Studies showed that delirium is phenomenologically similar in patients with or without dementia (although patients with dementia have more symptoms). Cole et al. (2002) reported that frequency of ten symptoms of delirium investigated by them in the elderly hospitalized patients was largely similar to each other in two delirium patient groups with and without dementia; only the rates of baseline psychomotor agitation and disorganized thinking and disorientation were higher in the group with dementia. Similar findings have been confirmed in some other studies despite some small differences in the distribution of symptoms. The authors concluded that delirium may not be phenomenologically different in patients with and without dementia (Levkoff et al. 1992; Trzepacz et al. 1998; Liptzin 1999; Margiotta et al. 2006).

Despite the above, when there is a sudden change in cognition or behaviour in an older patient, one should first consider delirium. Although it is very difficult to distinguish delirium and dementia, some clinical features can be guiding. Dementia presents insidiously with a gradual course of decline, while delirium presents as a sudden loss of global cognitive function. With delirium, attention and level of consciousness are reduced and fluctuating; with dementia, these cognitive domains typically remain intact until the advanced stages. A careful history is very important to diagnose dementia with or without delirium. Dementia frequently presents with a history of chronic, steady decline in memory and is associated with difficulties in social relationships, work and activities of daily life. It is of paramount importance to compare current mental status or cognition with their baseline according to information taken from relatives or carers. It should always be evaluated in favour of delirium when there are cognitive and behavioural changes which develop over hours or days in the older people. The resolution of symptoms following treatment of an acute illness or precipitating factors can sometimes retrospectively confirm the diagnosis of delirium.

In most demented patients, there is increased wandering, confusion and agitation in late afternoon and early evening (15.00–19.00 h). This is known as "sundowning syndrome" which can mimic the symptoms of hyperactive delirium (Drake et al.

1997). In cases where there is worsening in the second half of the day, it is important to get information from carers about previous pattern. In dementia this is usually chronic, and every day it tends to recur almost at the same time of the day. There could be a similar picture in delirium but in delirium symptoms fluctuate day to day both in timing and severity. Whether or not they have dementia, worsening of the symptoms in older patients in the late afternoon, it is best to query other symptoms of delirium and if in doubt investigate it as delirium.

It can be particularly difficult to distinguish delirium from Lewy body dementia (DLB) because some features, such as visual hallucinations and symptom fluctuation, are common to both. But in dementia with DLB, the history is usually longer (months or years) and there could be parkinsonian symptoms. Still, the safest clinical approach is to consider that all older people presenting with confusion have delirium until proved otherwise (Young and Inouye 2007).

### 3.4.2 Distinguishing Hypoactive Delirium and Depression

Delirium is misdiagnosed as depression in up to 40% of cases (Farrell and Ganzini 1995). Particularly, hypoactive delirium can mimic a retarded depression with slowed thinking, psychomotor slowing, sleep disturbance, irritability, decreased concentration and memory impairment. Cognitive symptoms like poor concentration, memory difficulties and delusions, hallucinations and sleep problems can be seen in elderly patients with psychotic depression. The history of the patient is important in such cases. The presentation in delirium tends to be more acute, whereas in depressive illness mood symptoms predominate and are pervasive and persistent. Depression usually has a history of previous episodes and no fluctuations. The level of consciousness and attention remains unaffected in depression. The predominance of depressive cognitions like ideas of guilt and worthlessness in depression is important in differential diagnosis.

### 3.4.3 Psychotic Disorders and Bipolar Disorder with Psychotic Features

Vivid hallucinations and delusions as described above are seen quite often in delirium. Language disturbances, abnormal behaviours and agitation can mask the diagnosis particularly in hyperactive delirium. There could be aggressive behaviour to an extent of homicide in agitated patients. This situation could be very uncomfortable for carers and clinical staff. This clinical picture can easily be mistaken as psychosis. On the other hand, in the elderly psychotic patients, there could sometimes be problems with consciousness and orientation which can be mistaken as "confusion". Some acute psychosis, especially with mania, is capable of producing delirium-like states. Hence, delirium must be distinguished from brief psychotic disorder, schizophrenia, schizophreniform disorder and other psychotic disorders, as well as from bipolar with psychotic features. In these cases, the history taken from relatives and other informants gains more importance. History about when and how symptoms started, episodes of psychosis or mood disorders are all important for diagnosis. In psychosis there is usually no impairment of awareness or attention. Schizophrenia is a longstanding illness which usually starts in young age typically with an insidious onset. Late-onset schizophrenia is very rare, and there is female gender and paranoid type predominance. Studies show that there are nearly 0.5% of people over 65 years with schizophrenia (Howard et al. 2000). Cognitive impairment is seen much less which is helpful in distinguishing from delirium. The sensorium is generally clear in schizophrenia and other psychotic disorders. Disturbance of thought and perception seen in delirium is often fragmentary, fluctuating and less complex than that seen in schizophrenia, in which delusions and hallucinations tend to be much more persistent and consistent. Delusions tend to be highly systematized, bizarre and uninfluenced by the environment. In contrast to psychoses, delusions in delirium are usually poorly systematized, fleeting and related to environmental stimuli. In schizophrenia it is usually auditory hallucinations that patients experience, whereas in delirium they are mostly visual or in other modalities. First-rank symptoms such as thought insertion, voices giving running commentary or talking to each other are not common in delirium.

Manic episodes can simulate hyperactive delirium, with diminished attention, agitation, rapid fluctuations and psychosis. Manic episodes in older adults often present with confusion, disorientation, distractibility and irritability rather than elevated, positive mood. Kraepelin in 1921 categorized mania into three types: acute, delusional and delirious. However, there is no clear consensus on the clinical characteristics associated with delirious mania or guidelines for treatment (Lee et al. 2012). Late-onset mania is more often secondary to or closely associated with other medical disorders, most commonly stroke, dementia or hyperthyroidism; it is also associated with medications including antidepressants, steroids, oestrogens and other agents with known central nervous system properties (Young et al. 1997). In the elderly patients, history and clinical presentation can help differentiate delirium from a manic episode. The history of depressive/manic episodes or elevated mood supports diagnosis of mania. Thought content is important as in depression cases. Increased self-esteem and grandiosity would suggest mania.

### 3.4.4 Other Disorders

Delirium associated with fear, anxiety and dissociative symptoms such as depersonalization also must be distinguished from acute stress disorder, anxiety and panic attacks. Acute stress disorder develops within the first month after exposure to a severely traumatic event such as rape, abuse, torture or war. One of the more common reasons for acute stress disorder in the elderly is witnessing the death of a friend or a loved one. Some arousal symptoms such as sleep disturbance, irritable behaviour and angry outbursts, hypervigilance, problems with concentration and exaggerated startle response can be seen in acute stress disorder and may be confused with delirium. Symptoms similar to delirium can be seen during an acute anxiety or panic attack. On the other hand, delirious people with reduced cognitive function and limited speech may exhibit anxiety that can manifest as an anxiety disorder. History from carers and relatives and querying other symptoms of these disorders would be helpful in differential diagnosis.

**Conclusion**

Delirium is a common and significant healthcare concern in elderly people. It is characterised by recent onset of fluctuating inattention and awareness, linked to several precipitating and aetiological factors. The existing research evidence suggests that delirium could be prevented in a lot of cases. However, it is reported to remain undiagnosed in more than half of clinical cases. History taken from relatives, clinical staff or carers is as valuable as a careful cognitive assessment. A rational approach would be to consider and investigate any new cognitive or behavioural problems in an older patient as delirium.

## References


American Psychiatric Association (2013) Diagnostic and statistical manual of mental disorders, 5th edn. American Psychiatric Association, Arlington, VA

Bergeron N, Dubois MJ, Dumont M et al (2001) Intensive Care Delirium Screening Checklist: evaluation of a new screening tool. Intensive Care Med 27(5):859–864

Blackburn HL, Benton AL (1957) Revised administration and scoring of the Digit Span Test. J Consult Psychol 21(2):139–114

Camus V, Gonthier R, Dubos G et al (2000) Etiologic and outcome profiles in hypoactive and hyperactive subtypes of delirium. J Geriatr Psychiatry Neurol 13(1):38–42

Cole M, Primeau F (1993) Prognosis of delirium in elderly hospital patients. Can Med Assoc J 149:41–46

Cole MG, McCusker J, Dendukuri N et al (2002) Symptoms of delirium among elderly medical inpatients with or without dementia. J Neuropsychiatry Clin Neurosci 14:167–175

Cornblatt BA, Risch NL, Faris G et al (1988) The continuous performance test, identical pairs version (CPT-IP): I. New findings about sustained attention in normal families. Psychiatry Res 26(2):223–238

Drake L, Drake V, Curwen J (1997) A new account of sundown syndrome. Nurs Stand 12(7):37–40

Ely EW, Margolin R, Francis J et al (2001) Evaluation of delirium in critically ill patients: validation of the Confusion Assessment Method for the Intensive Care Unit (CAM-ICU). Crit Care Med 29(7):1370–1379

Farrell KR, Ganzini L (1995) Misdiagnosing delirium as depression in medically ill elderly patients. Arch Intern Med 155:2459–2464

Fick D, Agostini JV, Inouye SK (2002) Delirium superimposed on dementia: a systematic review. J Am Geriatr Soc 50:1723–1732

Fick D, Lawrence F, Hodo D et al (2007) Recognizing delirium superimposed on dementia. Assessing nurses' knowledge using case vignettes. J Gerontol Nurs 34(6):40–47

Fong TG, Tulebaev SR, Inouye SK (2009) Delirium in elderly adults: diagnosis, prevention and treatment. Nat Rev Neurol 5(4):210–220

Gaudreau JD, Gagnon P, Harel F et al (2005) Fast, systematic, and continuous delirium assessment in hospitalized patients: the nursing delirium screening scale. J Pain Symptom Manage 29(4):368–375

Gottlieb G, Johnson J, Wanich C et al (1991) Delirium in the medically ill elderly: operationalizing the DSM-III criteria. Int Psychogeriatr 3:181–196

Howard R, Rabins PV, Seeman MV et al (2000) Late-onset schizophrenia and very-late-onset schizophrenia-like psychosis: an international consensus. Am J Psychiatry 157:172–178
Inouye SK (2006) Delirium in older persons. N Engl J Med 354:1157–1165
Inouye SK, Foreman MD, Mion LC et al (2001) Nurses recognition of delirium and its symptoms: comparison of nurse and researcher ratings. Arch Int Med 161:2467–2473
Inouye SK, van Dyck CH, Alessi CA et al (1990) Clarifying confusion: the confusion assessment method. Ann Intern Med 113:941–948
Inouye SK, Westendorp RG, Saczynski JS (2014) Delirium in elderly people. Lancet 383:911–922
Ismail Z, Rajji TK, Shulman KI (2010) Brief cognitive screening instruments: an update. Int J Geriatr Psychiatry 25:111–120
Justic M (2000) Does "ICU psychosis" really exist? Crit Care Nurse 20:28–37
Krahne D, Heymann A, Spies C (2006) How to monitor delirium in the ICU and why it is important. Clin Eff Nurs 9(Suppl 3):269–279
Lee BS, Huang SS, Hsu WY et al (2012) Clinical features of delirious mania: a series of five cases and a brief literature review. BMC Psychiatry 12:65. https://doi.org/10.1186/1471-244X-12-65
Levkoff S, Evans D, Liptzin B et al (1992) Delirium: the occurrence and persistence of symptoms among elderly hospitalized patients. Arch Intern Med 152:334–340
Lipowski ZJ (1980) A new look at organic brain syndromes. Am J Psychiatry 137:674–678
Lipowski ZJ (1983) Transient cognitive disorders (delirium, acute confusional states) in the elderly. Am J Psychiatry 140:1426–1436
Liptzin B (1999) What criteria should be used for the diagnosis of delirium? Dement Geriatr Cogn Disord 10:364–367
Liptzin B, Levkoff SE (1992) An empirical study of delirium subtypes. Br J Psychiatry 161:843–845
Marcantonio E, Ta T, Duthie E et al (2002) Delirium severity and psychomotor types: their relationship with outcomes after hip fracture repair. J Am Geriatr Soc 50:850–857
Margiotta A, Bianchetti A, Ranieri P et al (2006) Clinical characteristics and risk factors of delirium in demented and not demented elderly medical inpatients. J Nutr Health Aging 10(6):535–539
McCusker J, Cole M, Abrahamowicz M et al (2002) Delirium predicts 12-month mortality. Arch Intern Med 162:457–463
Meagher DJ, O'Hanlon D, O'Mahoney E (1996) The use of environmental strategy and psychotropic medication in the management of delirium. Br J Psychiatry 168(4):512–515
Meagher DJ, Trzepacz PT (1998) Delirium phenomenology illuminates pathophysiology, management, and course. J Geriatr Psychiatry Neurol 11(3):150–158
Michauda L, Bqlac C, Berneyb A et al (2007) Delirium: guidelines for general hospitals. J Psychosom Res 62:371–383
Neelon VJ, Champagne MT, Carlson JR et al (1996) The NEECHAM confusion scale: construction, validation, and clinical testing. Nurs Res 45(6):324–330
O'Keeffe ST, Lavan JN (1999) Clinical significance of delirium subtypes in older people. Age Ageing 28:115–119
O'Keeffe ST, Mulkerna EC, Nayeem K et al (2005) Use of serial mini-mental state examinations to diagnose and monitor delirium in elderly hospital patients. J Am Geriatr Soc 53:867–870
Otter H, Martin J, Basell K et al (2005) Validity and reliability of the DDS for severity of delirium in the ICU. Neurocrit Care 2:150–158
Pisani MA, Murphy TE, Van Ness PH et al (2007) Characteristics associated with delirium in older patients in a medical intensive care unit. Arch Intern Med 167:1629–1634
Rhodius-Meester HFMP, van Campen JPMC, Fung W et al (2013) Development and validation of the Informant Assessment of Geriatric Delirium Scale (I-AGeD): recognition of delirium in geriatric patients. Eur Geriatr Med 4:73–77
Ross C, Peyser C, Shapiro I et al (1991) Delirium: phenomenologic and etiologic subtypes. Int Psychogeriatr 3(2):135–147
Rudberg MA, Pompei P, Foreman MD et al (1997) The natural history of delirium in older hospitalised patients: a syndrome of heterogeneity. Age Ageing 26:169–174
Rummans TA, Evans JM, Krahn LE et al (1995) Delirium in elderly patients: evaluation and management. Mayo Clin Pract 70:989–998

Saxena S, Lawley D (2009) Delirium in the elderly: a clinical review. Postgrad Med J 85:405–413. https://doi.org/10.1136/pgmj.2008.072025
Siddiqi N, Horne AO, House AO et al (2006) Occurrence and outcome of delirium in medical inpatients; a systematic literature review. Age Ageing 35:350–364
Spronk PE, Riekerk B, Hofhuis J et al (2009) Occurrence of delirium is severely underestimated in the ICU during daily care. Intensive Care Med 35:1276–1280
Stagno D, Gibson C, Breitbart W (2004) The delirium subtypes: a review of prevalence, phenomenology, pathophysiology and treatment response. Palliat Support Care 2:171–179
Teasdale G (2014) Forty years on: updating the Glasgow Coma Scale. Nurs Times 110(42):12–16
Teasdale G, Jennett B (1974) Assessment of coma and impaired consciousness: a practical scale. Lancet 2:81–84
Treloar A, Macdonald J (1997) Outcome of delirium: part 2 clinical features of reversible cognitive dysfunction–are they the same as accepted definitions of delirium? Int J Geriatr Psychiatry 12(6):614–618
Trzepacz PT (1994) The neuropathogenesis of delirium: a need to focus our research. Psychosomatics 35:374–391
Trzepacz PT (1999) Update on neuropathogenesis of delirium. Dement Geriatr Cogn Disord 10:330–334
Trzepacz PT, Mittal D, Torres R et al (2001) Validation of the delirium rating scale-revised-98: comparison with the delirium rating scale and the cognitive test for delirium. J Neuropsychiatry Clin Neurosci 13(2):229–242
Trzepacz PT, Mulsant BH, Dew MA et al (1998) Is delirium different when it occurs in dementia? A study using the Delirium Rating Scale. J Neuropsychiatry Clin Neurosci 10:199–204
Webster R, Holroyd S (2000) Prevalence of psychotic symptoms in delirium. Psychosomatics 41(6):519–522
World Health Organization (1992) The tenth revision of the International Classification of Diseases and Related Health Problems (ICD–10). WHO, Geneva
Young J, Inouye SK (2007) Delirium in older people. BMJ 334:842–846. https://doi.org/10.1136/bmj.39169.706574.AD
Young RC, Moline M, Kleyman F (1997) Estrogen replacement therapy and late life mania. Am J Geriatr Psychiatry 5(2):179–181

# Delirium Superimposed on Dementia

# 4

Ahmet Turan Isik

Delirium is an acute potentially life-threatening condition characterized by inattention, generalized cognitive impairments, and disturbances in consciousness mainly affecting elderly inpatients (Steis and Fick 2012). In contrast, dementia, the most common form being Alzheimer's disease (AD), is characterized by insidious onset, normal level of consciousness, and a chronic or slowly progressive irreversible decline in cognitive function (Isik 2010). Increasing numbers of demented elderly patients are hospitalized and are at increased risk of developing delirium, and delirium occurs in most of them (Steis and Fick 2012), and a chronic delirious state might be observed in advanced demented elderly patients (Moraga and Rodriguez-Pascual 2007).

Delirium might worsen the clinical course, cognitive decline, and activities of daily living and might be associated with exaggeration of behavioral and psychological symptoms of dementia, cerebrovascular disease in patients with neurodegenerative dementias, prolonged hospitalization, rehospitalization within 30 days, nursing home placement, and death in elderly demented patients (Fong et al. 2009, 2012; Hasegawa et al. 2013; Fick et al. 2013). It was also reported that delirium was associated with high risk of institutionalization (fivefold) and mortality (twofold) at 1-year follow-up in elderly patients with dementia (Morandi et al. 2014) and along with worsening of existing cognitive decline (Gross et al. 2012; Davis et al. 2017), when compared to delirium alone. On the other hand, preexisting dementia is accepted one of the factors related to prolonged and refractory course of delirium or late response to therapy (Boettger et al. 2014).

Therefore, delirium that occurs in patients with dementia is referred to as delirium superimposed on dementia (DSD). DSD is diagnosed when an acute change in mental status, such as a fluctuating course, inattention, and either disorganized thinking or changes in consciousness, is observed in elderly patients with dementia

A.T. Isik, M.D.
Unit for Aging Brain and Dementia, Department of Geriatric Medicine, Faculty of Medicine, Dokuz Eylul University, Izmir, 35340 Turkey
e-mail: atisik@yahoo.com



A.T. Isik, G.T. Grossberg (eds.), *Delirium in Elderly Patients*,
https://doi.org/10.1007/978-3-319-65239-9_4

(Fick et al. 2002). Although delirium and dementia are two distinct common geriatric syndromes, they can present with similar symptoms, and dementia is generally considered a major risk factor for delirium (Hasegawa et al. 2013; Inouye 2006). In addition, although it is known that there is a strong physiopathological and clinical interrelationship between both syndromes, the relationship between delirium and dementia could not be clarified exactly (Young and Inouye 2007).

The prevalence of delirium in elderly patients was reported as 1–2%, while it was reported increasingly up to 22% in elderly demented patients (de Lange et al. 2012). The prevalence of delirium superimposed on dementia reportedly increased up to 89% in community and hospital populations (Fick et al. 2002). Hospitalization is an important factor for development of DSD in older patients (Fong et al. 2012), when approximately 80% of elderly patients with dementia hospitalized experience delirium, and mortality ratio within 1 year of the delirium episode was reported as 24–76% (McCusker et al. 2001a), and dementia may increase the risk for development of delirium up to 40% (McNicoll et al. 2003). In spite of the poor outcomes and high prevalence of DSD, little is known about the course of disease in demented elderly inpatients. Even though dementia is usually exclusion criteria for delirium studies, the prevalence of DSD is extremely high in both community dwelling and hospitalized elderly patients (13–19% and 40–89%, respectively) and associated with higher costs and utilization compared to dementia and delirium alone (Fick et al. 2005, 2013).

## 4.1 Why Is the Delirium Commonly Encountered in Elderly Patients with Dementia?

The delirium and dementia are age-related conditions, geriatric syndromes, and the prevalence of both increases with age. Delirium is not only common in demented patients (OR 5.3) (Francis et al. 1990), but its prevalence also changes according to type of dementia. In a prospective cohort study, that 206 demented outpatients were evaluated, delirium was presented in 19.4% of the patients; however, it was determined that the prevalence of delirium varies with each dementia type: 14.7% for AD, 34.4% for vascular dementia (VaD), and 31.8% for dementia of Lewy body (DLB), and the prevalence of DSD was related to cerebrovascular disease (Hasegawa et al. 2013).

Delirium is encountered four to five times more frequent in a demented patient; nevertheless, what is more remarkable is that recognition and treatment of DSD are less likely than are the delirium without dementia (Fong et al. 2012; Inouye 2006). This could be termed as DSD paradox. The underlining reason for the basis of this paradox is the similar symptomatology commonly shared by both diseases. So, the diagnosis and the treatment might delay due to the fact that acute mental changes in elderly patients are overlooked, misdiagnosed, or attributed to natural course and behavioral and psychological symptoms of dementia (BPSD) (Landreville et al. 2013), especially in DLB in which among the core features are fluctuating cognition and recurrent visual hallucinations (Gore et al. 2015). When DSD could not be diagnosed and treated on time, it could be an important problem that may have life-threatening complications, in dementia practice.

Current evidence supported that delirium is significantly associated with developing cognitive impairment and dementia, increases the risk of death, and accelerates cognitive impairments in patients with dementia, while preexisting dementia plays an important role in occurrence, severity, and persistence of delirium (Voyer et al. 2011); furthermore, severity of dementia is an independent risk factor for delirium (Robertson et al. 1998). According to cognitive impairment, Davis et al. reported that DSD is associated with accelerated cognitive decline beyond that expected for delirium or the pathologic process itself, and these suggest that additional unmeasured pathologic processes specifically relate to delirium. Besides, it was also reported that delirium appears to act independently and multiplicatively to the neuropathologic processes of classic dementia (Davis et al. 2017). In addition, it was reported that delirium might represent early or prodromal DLB at least in some cases and might play a role as a diagnostic marker for DLB since both diseases share many more similar clinical and physiopathological features (Gore et al. 2015). Shortly, it should always be kept in mind each disease can potentialize the development of another in dementia.

## 4.2 Clinical Features

Delirium is acute confusional state; however, dementia is chronically confusional state (Hanson and Galvez-Jimenez 2004; Wilber 2006). Clinically, in the patients with DSD, the overlapping features of both diseases may confuse the development of clinical diagnosis. The deleterious effect of DSD, in a cohort study, explained as the symptoms of delirium is predominated than that of dementia as irrelevant to severity of cognitive impairment (Trzepacz et al. 1998). On the other hand, due to the prior cognitive dysfunction, most of symptoms of delirium are exacerbated, particularly attentional impairment, disorientation, disorganization of thought, and memory impairment in patients with DSD (Boettger et al. 2014), and cognitive status of patients also plays a role in recovery of the delirium (Chong et al. 2015).

Even though the clinical features and course of both delirium and dementia, theoretically, seem like enough to differentiate from each other, this, practically, cannot be possible any particular moment in time, since differential diagnosis needs close monitoring for disease progression. In addition, Gore et al. also reported that elderly patients presenting with delirium should be followed up and observed for occurrence of dementia especially for DLB (Gore et al. 2015).

Apart from general features of delirium without dementia (DWD) in the elderly, the clinical features of the DSD include (Boettger et al. 2014; Chong et al. 2015; Leonard et al. 2014):

- The deterioration in the level of consciousness is more severe (OD 4.56): this may be a remarkable feature of the DSD.
- The impairment in the cognitive functions/domain is more severe (OD 1.97 to 2.85), especially in the ability to maintain and shift attention and thought disorder/speech.

- Delirium symptoms are more severe intensity.
- The severity of hallucinations, delusions, psychomotor abnormality, or sleep–wake cycle disturbances is similar to those with DWD.
- Remarkable presentation of delirium is hypoactive delirium in the palliative care.
- Recovery of cognitive symptoms is slower, and duration of the disease is longer.
- Late response to treatment.
- Delirium may be first sign of cognitive impairment/dementia.

As mentioned before, the diagnosis of DSD requires a collateral history obtained from the informant, but often a lack of individuals who can report an acute change from baseline may delay diagnosis or result in delirium being missed, leading to worse outcomes (Kakuma et al. 2003). Therefore, it is important that combining simple and brief assessments of attention and arousal for accurate diagnoses of DSD independent of the informant is appealing in this setting where time is limited and an informant is not always immediately available. For this purpose, Richardson et al. developed an evaluation by combining arousal–attention assessment to detect DSD (93% correctly classified, sensitivity 94%, specificity 92%, AUROC 0.98). It has brief yet high diagnostic accuracy even in dementia and might have major clinical utility for diagnosing DSD (Richardson et al. 2017). In addition, since DSD is a complex clinical condition, which can be resulted in very poor outcomes, and the lack of standardization in the assessment of DSD may have potential significant clinical and research implications, iDelirium group (www.idelirium.org) reported descriptions of its presentation and associated clinical findings and the insufficiency of current diagnostic assessment tools as a framework. In this report, as shown in Fig. 4.1, the authors pointed out that a key feature of a reliable reference standard will improve the ability to clinically diagnose DSD in facility-based patients and research studies (Morandi et al. 2017).

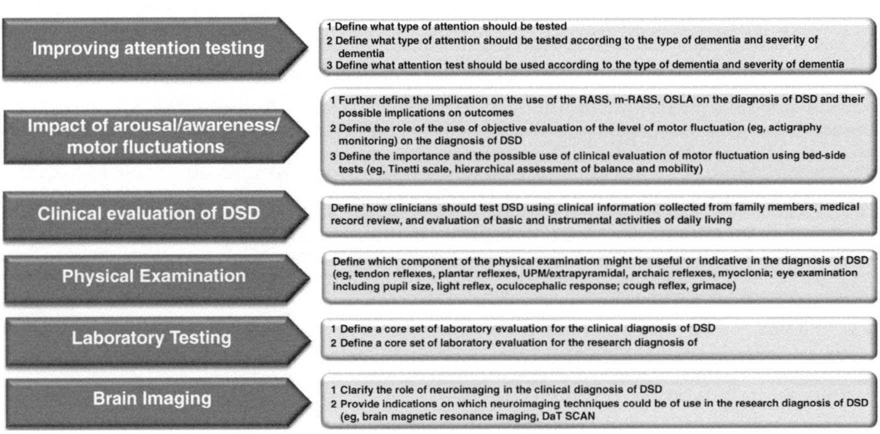


**Fig. 4.1** iDelirium group's report for Improving to Diagnoses of DSD (Morandi et al. 2017). *DSD* dementia superimposed dementia

On the other hand, in differential diagnosis of DSD, progression of the dementia and psychological symptoms of dementia (BPSD) should be considered (Morandi et al. 2017). The fact that delirium decreases activities of daily living and exacerbates BPSD in preexisting dementia should also be kept in mind.

## 4.3 Physiopathological Mechanisms in Delirium Superimposed on Dementia

There are some sharing putative pathophysiological mechanisms as well as some clinical features between delirium and dementia. Most prominent among these mechanisms are the phenomena of reduced cerebral cholinergic neurotransmission, systemic inflammation, neuroinflammation, blood–brain barrier impairment, and reversible decrease in flow velocity and in cerebral blood flow (Leonard et al. 2014; Caplan et al. 2014). In addition, DSD is also associated, as in non-demented patients, with deregulation of neurotransmitter systems (Cerejeira et al. 2010).

According to the neuronal aging hypothesis of delirium, in the elderly patients, especially with dementia, neuropathologic changes, resulting in overactivated microglia, render such patients more vulnerable to the effects of systemic inflammation. Due to the vulnerability of the elderly with dementia, relatively minor infections may trigger an episode of delirium (Leonard et al. 2014). Acetylcholine inhibits the microglial activity in the central nervous system (Pavlov et al. 2009). In the event of cholinergic deficiency such as in aging brain, dementia, or usage of anticholinergic medications, microglia overactivates. This may explain the predisposing vulnerability to delirium in the patient with dementia, where systemic inflammation such as infections may cross the blood–brain barrier. This could explain the persistence of some delirium symptoms in association with neuroinflammation and secondary neurodegeneration, even after the apparently successful treatment of infection (Leonard et al. 2014).

Apart from these mechanisms, it should be known that the cognitive reserve of elderly patients with DSD may account for changes in vulnerability to age-related and pathologic brain changes in manifesting cognitive symptoms (Chong et al. 2015; Tucker and Stern 2011).

## 4.4 Management

It is important to develop primary and secondary prevention and therefore close contact with the patient. Ensuring adequate vision, hearing, nutrition, hydration, and sleep; informing caregivers about early symptoms of delirium; mobilizing the patient as early as possible; and managing the pain are strongly recommended. Besides, clinicians must identify the real underlying medical conditions such as the use of restraints or new medication. Since delirium often results from a lot of interaction of factors in elderly patients, all those factors should be checked and eradicated. Firstly, common causes in elderly, such as malnutrition, pressure ulcers, urinary incontinence, polypharmacy, chronic pain, falls, electrolyte imbalance, fecal impaction or urinary retention, hypoxia, dehydration, poor vision and hearing, and environmental factors, should be assessed. Non-pharmacological approaches are the first-line strategy. Especially in patients with DSD, monitoring predisposing and precipitating factors, maximizing family support, orienting communication (placing clocks, calendars, photo in the room), mobility, minimizing medication use, ensuring adequate hydration, and attending to sensory needs such as vision and hearing impairment are very important at this stage (Isik 2014; Kalish et al. 2014; Inouye et al. 2014).

Suicidality, violence potential, fall risk, wandering risk, and inadvertent self-harm risk should all be assessed with appropriate measures taken to ensure safety. The use of restraints should be minimized as they may increase agitation and hence decrease safety (Hofmann and Schneider 2007). The patient should be stabilized in a quiet room if possible. If TV or radio sounds seem to increase anxiety or agitation, then these should be avoided. Activity—such as walking, sitting up in a chair, and active or passive range of motion exercises—should be promoted and scheduled with alternating rest periods (Morandi et al. 2015). In a study, it was demonstrated that patients with DSD in the intervention group developed significantly less delirium than those in the usual care group and had significant improvement in orientation scores on the MMSE (Inouye et al. 1999). Another study showed that dementia status was associated with delirium but did not indicate whether influences of the non-pharmacological interventions were more or less important for patients with DSD (McCusker et al. 2001b). Since the results of studies were confusing, future intervention studies are greatly needed in comparing outcomes in patients with delirium, DSD, and dementia alone.

Initial screening test for detecting etiology of delirium as in all patients with delirium should be included. Further investigations based on clues from history, physical examination, and previous results are indicated if initial analyses fail (Inouye 1998).

If non-pharmacological interventions are insufficient, pharmacologic therapy should be implemented. Antipsychotics have been the medication of choice in the treatment of delirium. However, there are no Food and Drug Administration (FDA)-approved medications for delirium, and clinicians must be aware that these drugs for the treatment of delirium can have significant side effects. Thus, the drug should be given in the lowest possible dose for the shortest duration. Also, pharmacologic agents should be reserved for patients with severe agitation, which may result in the interruption of essential medical therapies (e.g., intubation, intra-aortic balloon pumps, dialysis catheters) or which may endanger the safety of the patient, other patients, or staff (Inouye et al. 2014; Hofmann and Schneider 2007).

Haloperidol is considered to be the first preferred agent for the pharmacological management of delirium, with its high potency and minimal anticholinergic and cardiovascular side effects. It is recommended to start haloperidol at a dose of 1.0 mg orally or parenterally and to repeat the dose every 20–30 min until the patient is calm enough. Vital signs should be checked before repeating each dose. Subsequently, a maintenance dose of one half of the loading dose should be administered in divided doses over the next 24 h, with tapering doses over the next few days (Rana and Morren 2013; Kennedy 2003).

Regarding the newer antipsychotic medications in the treatment of delirium, it was demonstrated that risperidone, olanzapine, and quetiapine were as effective and safe as haloperidol (Yoon et al. 2013). In addition, it was reported that olanzapine might reduce the incidence but increase the duration and severity of delirium (Larsen et al. 2010). Besides these reports, it is essential to keep in mind that these atypical antipsychotic drugs were issued a black box warning by FDA due to their 1.6–1.7 times higher death rate when compared to placebo in patients with DSD (Hofmann and Schneider 2007). Therefore, in patients with DSD, antipsychotic drugs should be used carefully since polypharmacy and multiple comorbid conditions are common in the elderly.

There are some drugs for the treatment of delirium, which are recommended in different types of dementia. When using antipsychotic drugs in Lewy body dementia and/or Parkinson's disease, agitation and confusion may increase (NICE 2010). In these cases benzodiazepines may be recommended. Benzodiazepines also are used in cases of withdrawal syndromes from alcohol and sedative-hypnotic drugs, agitation due to neuroleptic malignant syndrome, and catatonia or severe extrapyramidal reactions. Lorazepam is the first choice with a starting dose of 0.5–1.0 mg in geriatric population. It does not have active metabolites and has advantages such as its parenteral form and relatively less half-life which is approximately 10–15 h (Rana and Morren 2013; Vardi and Harrington 2014). Cholinergic deficit may play a role in the development of DSD, but there isn't enough evidence to demonstrate that acetylcholinesterase inhibitors (AchEIs) are effective in the prevention or treatment (Gamberini et al. 2009). Nevertheless, it was reported that AchEIs might benefit patients with delirium superimposed on Lewy body dementia and/or Parkinson's disease (Tabet and Howard 2009. In our clinical practice, AchEI therapy is sensible to maintain for patients with dementia undergoing medical procedure, but routine prescription of prophylactic AchEIs cannot be recommended.

Melatonin plays a central role in the regulation of the sleep–wake cycle, which is frequently disrupted in delirium. In addition, alterations of melatonin metabolism may be effective in the development of delirium. According to this, it was demonstrated that 0.5 mg/day of melatonin for up to 14 days was associated with lower delirium risk compared with placebo, and it was recommended that nightly melatonin could have potential protective effect for delirium in elderly patients (Al-Aama et al. 2011). The use of melatonin also to treat and to prevent DSD is considered (Roden and Simmons 2014).

Valproate, ondansetron, gabapentin, and anti-inflammatory drugs may be used to treat delirium with or without dementia, but further investigations are required to explain their efficiency.

In conclusion, it is clearly obvious that delirium and dementia in an elderly patient have a reciprocal relationship. While delirium might be associated with increased BPSD, worsening in natural course dementia, cerebrovascular disease prolonged hospitalization, rehospitalization within 30 days, nursing home placement, and mortality in elderly patients with dementia, preexisting dementia is also associated with prolonged and refractory course of delirium or late response to therapy. So, preventive approaches for DSD and early diagnoses and management should not be left out for elderly patients with DSD.

## References

Al-Aama T, Brymer C, Gutmanis I et al (2011) Melatonin decreases delirium in elderly patients: a randomized, placebo-controlled trial. Int J Geriatr Psychiatry 26:687–694

Boettger S, Jenewein J, Breitbart W (2014) Delirium in advanced age and dementia: a prolonged refractory course of delirium and lower functional status. Palliat Support Care 13(4):1113–1121

Caplan GA, Lan ZZ, Newton L et al (2014) Transcranial doppler to measure cerebral blood flow in delirium superimposed on dementia. A cohort study. JAMDA 15:355e360

Cerejeira J, Firmino H, Vaz-Serra A et al (2010) The neuroinflammatory hypothesis of delirium. Acta Neuropathol 119:737–754

Chong E, Tay L, Chong MS (2015) Identifying phenomenological differences and recovery of cognitive and non-cognitive symptomatology among delirium superimposed upon dementia patients (DsD) versus those without dementia (DaD) in an acute geriatric care setting. Int Psychogeriatr 9:1–11

Davis HJ, Muniz-Terrera G, Keage HAD et al (2017) Association of delirium with cognitive decline in late life: a neuropathologic study of 3 population-based cohort studies. J Am Med Assoc Psychiatry 74:244–251

Francis J, Martin D, Kapoor WN (1990) A prospective study of delirium in hospitalized elderly. JAMA 263(8):1097–1101

Fick D, Agostini JV, Inouye SK (2002) Delirium superimposed on dementia: a systematic review. J Am Geriatr Soc 50:1723–1732

Fick DM, Kolanowski A, Waller JL et al (2005) Delirium superimposed on dementia in a community-dwelling managed care population: a 3-year retrospective study of occurrence, costs, and utilization. J Gerontol 60A(6):748–753

Fick DM, Steis MR, Waller JL et al (2013) Delirium superimposed on dementia is associated with prolonged length of stay and poor outcomes in hospitalized older adults. J Hosp Med 8:500–505

Fong TG, Jones RN, Shi P et al (2009) Delirium accelerates cognitive decline in Alzheimer disease. Neurology 72:1570–1575

Fong TG, Jones RN, Marcantonio ER et al (2012) Adverse outcomes after hospitalization and delirium in persons with Alzheimer disease. Ann Intern Med 156(12):848–856

Gamberini M, Bolliger D, Lurati Buse GA et al (2009) Rivastigmine for the prevention of postoperative delirium in elderly patients undergoing elective cardiac surgery—a randomized controlled trial. Crit Care Med 37(5):1762–1768

Gore RL, Vardy ERLC, O'Brien JT (2015) Delirium and dementia with Lewy bodies: distinct diagnoses or part of the same spectrum? J Neurol Neurosurg Psychiatry 86(1):50–59

Gross AL, Jones RN, Habtemariam DA et al (2012) Delirium and long-term cognitive trajectory among persons with dementia. Arch Intern Med 172:1324–1331

Hanson MR, Galvez-Jimenez N (2004) Management of dementia and acute confusional states in the perioperative period. Neurol Clin 22:413–422

Hasegawa N, Hashimoto M, Yuuki S et al (2013) Prevalence of delirium among outpatients with dementia. Int Psychogeriatr 25(11):1877–1883

Hofmann M, Schneider D (2007) Practice guidelines for the treatment of patients with delirium. In: Skolnik NS (ed) Current clinical practice: essential practice guidelines in primary care. Humana Press, Totowa, NJ, pp 341–349

Inouye SK (1998) Delirium in hospitalized older patients. Clin Geriatr Med 14(4):745–765

Inouye SK (2006) Delirium in older persons. N Engl J Med 354:1157–1165

Inouye SK, Bogardus ST, Charpentier PA et al (1999) A multicomponent intervention to prevent delirium in hospitalized older patients. N Engl J Med 340:669–676
Inouye SK, Westendorp RGJ, Saczynski JS (2014) Delirium in elderly people. Lancet 383:911–922
Isik AT (2010) Late onset Alzheimer's disease in older people. Clin Interv Aging 5:307–311
Isik AT (2014) Geriatrik Olgularda Deliryum/Delirium in The Elderly. İzmir Guven Kitap, Izmir, Turkey. isbn:978-605-60355
Kakuma R, du Fort GG, Arsenault L et al (2003) Delirium in older emergency department patients discharged home: effect on survival. J Am Geriatr Soc 51:443–450
Kalish VB, Gillham JE, Unwin BK (2014) Delirium in older persons: evaluation and management. Am Fam Physician 90(3):150–158
Kennedy GJ (2003) Dementia. In: Cassel CK, Leipzig RM, Cohen HJ, Larson EB, Meier DE (eds) Geriatric medicine: an evidence-based approach, 4th edn. Springer, New York, pp 1079–1093
Landreville P, Voyer P, Carmichael PH (2013) Relationship between delirium and behavioral symptoms of dementia. Int Psychogeriatr 25:635–643
de Lange E, Verhaak PF, van der Meer K (2012) Prevalence, presentation and prognosis of delirium in older people in the population, at home and in long-term care: a review. Int J Geriatr Psychiatry 28:127–134
Larsen KA, Kelly SE, Stern TA (2010) Administration of olanzapine to prevent postoperative delirium in elderly joint-replacement patients: a randomized, controlled trial. Psychosomatics 51(5):409–418
Leonard MM, Agar M, Spiller JA (2014) Delirium diagnostic and classification challenges in palliative care: subsyndromal delirium, comorbid delirium-dementia, and psychomotor subtypes. J Pain Symptom Manag 48:199–214
McCusker J, Cole M, Abrahamowicz M et al (2001a) Environmental risk factors for delirium in hospitalized older people. J Am Geriatr Soc 49:1327–1334
McCusker J, Cole M, Dendukuri N (2001b) Delirium in older medical inpatients & subsequent cognitive & functional status: a prospective study. CMAJ 165:575–583
McNicoll L, Pisani MA, Zhang Y et al (2003) Delirium in the intensive care unit: occurrence and clinical course in older patients. J Am Geriatr Soc 51:591–598
Moraga AV, Rodriguez-Pascual C (2007) Accurate diagnosis of delirium in elderly patients. Curr Opin Psychiatry 20:262–267
Morandi A, Davis D, Fick DM et al (2014) Delirium superimposed on dementia strongly predicts worse outcomes in older rehabilitation inpatients. JAMDA 15(2014):349–354
Morandi A, Lucchi E, Turco R et al (2015) Delirium superimposed on dementia: A quantitative and qualitative evaluation of patient experience. J Psychosom Res 79(4):281–287
Morandi A, Davis D, Bellelli G et al (2017) The diagnosis of delirium superimposed on dementia: an emerging challenge. J Am Med Dir Assoc 18(1):12–18
National Institute for Health and Care Excellence (2010) Delirium: diagnosis, prevention and management
Pavlov VA, Parrish WR, Rosas-Ballina M et al (2009) Brain acetylcholinesterase activity controls systemic cytokine levels through the cholinergic antiinflammatory pathway. Brain Behav Immun 23:41e45
Rana AQ, Morren JA (2013) Delirium, neurological emergencies in clinical practice. Springer, London, pp 15–23
Richardson SJ, Davis DHJ, Bellelli G et al (2017) Detecting delirium superimposed on dementia: diagnostic accuracy of a simple combined arousal and attention testing procedure. Int Psychogeriatr 31:1–9
Robertson B, Blennow K, Gottfries CG et al (1998) Delirium in dementia. Int J Geriatr Psychiatry 13:49–56
Roden M, Simmons BB (2014) Delirium superimposed on dementia and mild cognitive impairment. Postgrad Med 126(6):129–137
Steis MR, Fick DM (2012) Delirium superimposed on dementia: accuracy of nurse documentation. J Gerontol Nurs 38:32–42

Tabet N, Howard R (2009) Pharmacological treatment for the prevention of delirium: review of current evidence. Int J Geriatr Psychiatry 24(10)

Trzepacz PT, Mulsant BH, Dew MA (1998) Is delirium different when it occurs in dementia? A study using the delirium rating scale. J Neuropsychiatr Clin Neurosci 10:199–204

Tucker AM, Stern Y (2011) Cognitive research imaging. Curr Alzheimer Res 8:354–360

Vardi K, Harrington CJ (2014) Delirium: treatment and prevention (part 2). R I Med J 97(6):24–28

Voyer P, Richard S, Doucet L (2011) Factors associated with delirium severity among older persons with dementia. J Neurosci Nurs 43:62–69

Wilber ST (2006) Altered mental status in older emergency department patients. Emerg Med Clin North Am 24:299–316

Young J, Inouye SK (2007) Delirium in older people. BMJ 334:842–846

Yoon HJ, Park KM, Choi WJ et al (2013) Efficacy and safety of haloperidol versus atypical antipsychotic medications in the treatment of delirium. BMJ Psychiatry 13:240;1–11

# Approach to the Elderly Patient with Delirium: Geriatrician's Perspective

5

Esra Ates Bulut and Ahmet Turan Isik

Delirium is an acute alteration of cognition hallmarked by disorganized thinking and inattention and a major health-care concern in countries with aging populations (Siddiqi et al. 2006). Delirium is a potent and well-recognized indicator of health-care quality across many settings (Inouye et al. 2014) and is an independent risk factor for length of hospitalization, increased functional impairment, medical complications (e.g., urinary incontinence, falls, decubitus ulcers), and admission to a nursing home (Siddiqi et al. 2006). Although delirium is associated with poor outcomes and is expensive, it remains hard to recognize (Inouye 2006). The American Psychiatric Association's *Diagnostic and Statistical Manual*, 5th edition, key diagnostic features include disturbance in attention (reduced ability to direct, focus, sustain, and shift attention) and awareness; fluctuating course during the day; an additional disturbance in cognition (memory deficit, disorientation, language, visuospatial ability, or perception); evidence from the history, physical examination, or laboratory findings that the disturbance is caused by a medical condition; substance intoxication or withdrawal; or medication side effect (Inouye et al. 1990; American Psychiatric Association 2013). Supportive features include disturbance in sleep–wake cycle, perceptual disturbances (hallucinations or illusions), delusions, psychomotor disturbance (hypoactivity or hyperactivity), inappropriate behavior, and emotional lability (Inouye 2006). Furthermore, that delirium occurs in older adults with dementia is also complex clinical conditions as well as delirium alone, in geriatric practice. This condition is referred to as delirium superimposed on dementia (DSD), and it is more responsible increased walking dependence,

E.A. Bulut, M.D.
Department of Geriatric Medicine, Faculty of Medicine, Dokuz Eylul University, 35340 Izmir, Turkey

A.T. Isik, M.D. (✉)
Unit for Aging Brain and Dementia, Department of Geriatric Medicine, Faculty of Medicine, Dokuz Eylul University, 35340 Izmir, Turkey
e-mail: atisik@yahoo.com



A.T. Isik, G.T. Grossberg (eds.), *Delirium in Elderly Patients*,
https://doi.org/10.1007/978-3-319-65239-9_5

institutionalization, and mortality along with worsening of existing cognitive decline than delirium alone (Davis et al. 2017; Gross et al. 2012; Morandi et al. 2014; Richardson et al. 2017). DSD is evaluated as a separate subtitle (Chap. 4) in this book.

## 5.1 Epidemiology

The prevalence of delirium in the community is 1–2% but increases in the setting of general hospital admissions to 6–56% (Fong et al. 2009), with the higher prevalence associated with increased age and increased severity of medical illness (Bucht et al. 1999). Postoperative prevalence of delirium in elderly patients ranges from 9 to 87%, and elderly patients with dementia and those undergoing cardiothoracic, emergency orthopedic procedures, vascular surgery, or cataract removal are at higher risk for developing delirium (Fong et al. 2009; Saxena and Lawley 2009). In addition to this, delirium is seen 8–17% in older emergency department patients (Han et al. 2009). The frequency in the emergency department is not low to underestimate.

## 5.2 Risk Factors

Risks for delirium can be divided into predisposing and precipitating factors (Inouye et al. 1993). Predisposing factors such as age, visual impairment, hearing impairment, severe illness, and cognitive impairment are the baseline vulnerabilities of an older person. In addition, geriatric syndromes, such as dementia, depression, malnutrition, pressure ulcers, urinary incontinence, polypharmacy, chronic pain, and falls, are associated with delirium. Precipitating factors are the acute and noxious insults experienced by an older person such as infection, metabolic derangement, or surgery (Inouye and Charpentier 1996). The development of delirium results from a complex interrelationship between predisposing and precipitating factors. These risk factors are shown in Table 5.1 (Isik 2014; Kalish et al. 2014; Soysal et al. 2015).

It is of special importance that elderly patients undergoing surgery have a high risk of postoperative delirium which is associated with both short- and long-term adverse events. The risk is higher in patients who have emergency surgery than those who have elective surgery. It could be seen in all kinds of surgery including cataract. However, it is most commonly seen after cardiovascular and hip fracture surgeries. Major postoperative complications, loss of functional independence, falls, increased length of hospital stay, discharge to long-term care, and death were reported as adverse outcome measures. Therefore, preoperative geriatric assessment is essential in older patients, because it not only informs the risk/benefit ratio for surgery but also identifies high-risk patients for early preoperative interventions and planning of intra- and postoperative care (Ansaloni et al. 2010).

**Table 5.1** Risk factors for delirium (adapted from Isik 2014; Inouye et al. 1993; Inouye and Charpentier 1996; Kalish et al. 2014; Soysal et al. 2015)

| Predisposing factors | Precipitating factors |
|---|---|
| Age (older than 65 years) | Dehydration |
| Male sex | Fracture |
| Chronic pain | Hypoxia |
| History of baseline lung, liver, kidney, heart, or brain disease | Infections |
| Terminal illness | Ischemia |
| Alcoholism | Medications |
| Dementia | Metabolic derangement |
| Depression | Poor nutrition |
| Elder abuse | Severe illness |
| Falls | Shock |
| History of delirium | Surgery |
| Malnutrition | Uncontrolled pain |
| Polypharmacy | Urinary retention |
| Pressure ulcers | Stool retention |
| Sensory impairment | Sleep deprivation/constipation |
| Inactivity | Hypo/hyperglycemia |
| Traumatic brain injury | Corticosteroids |
| Poor functional status | Intensive care unit setting |
| Social isolation | |

## 5.3 Clinical Presentations and Diagnosis

Delirium may occur within days or sometimes hours and the clinical features fluctuate during the day. The disturbance is generally caused by a medical condition, substance intoxication, or medication side effect. There are three core symptom domains including a "cognitive" domain, a "higher-level thinking" domain (language and thought process), and a "circadian" domain (sleep–wake cycle and motor behavior) (Caraceni and Grassi 2011).

Clinical presentation of delirium can range from frank somnolence to more awake and alert states. Patients may manifest clinical findings of obvious confusion with inappropriate response to questions. Sometimes, patients can focus initially but are distractible, impersistent, or perseverative on bedside evaluation. Restlessness, disheveled appearance, picking, and talking out loud when alone in the clinic may be observed. Generally, motor behavior abnormalities may also be observed in the patients. Delirium may be presented with hypoactive, hyperactive, and mixed subtypes according to these behaviors. The features of hypoactive delirium are psychomotor slowing, decreased in oral intake, limited engagement with the environment, inconvenience, tearfulness, withdrawal, and apathy. On the contrary, agitation, restlessness, anxiety, disinhibition, disordered thinking, and perceptual disturbances of hallucinations and delusions are usually seen in the hyperactive subtype of delirium. Hyperactive delirium may be associated with patient and staff injury and is more responsive to pharmacologic treatment. Hypoactive delirium is associated with a worse outcome. Cognitive and behavioral changes frequently fluctuate and follow a diurnal pattern. Assessment during periods of more lucid behavior can lead to the conclusion that patients are cognitively intact leading to the diagnosis being delayed or overlooked. In mixed delirium, patients often fluctuate between hypoactive and hyperactive subtypes of the disease (Isik 2014; Caraceni and Grassi 2011).

Standardized tools may help to efficiently and accurately diagnose delirium. The Confusion Assessment Method (CAM) is a widely used delirium screening instrument based on the DSM-III-R criteria (Inouye et al. 1990). The test is quick, easy, and inexpensive. Screening for delirium is positive if symptoms are acute at onset and have a fluctuating course, and the patient exhibits inattentiveness plus disorganized thought or altered consciousness (Inouye et al. 1990). Besides the CAM-ICU instrument has been developed and validated for identification of delirium in the intensive care unit (Ely et al. 2001).

## 5.4 Prevention and Treatment

Prevention is the main topic at the management of the delirium in the geriatric practice. It is important to health-care professionals to perform preventative strategies for patients at high risk and be aware of the potential for each single older adult to develop delirium, at the beginning. It should be kept in mind that early recognition and improving or reducing risk factors can significantly impact on the frequency of delirium in acute care settings (Soysal et al. 2015; Tomlinson et al. 2017).

*Non-pharmacologic interventions*: Primary prevention of delirium is the most effective strategy to reduce delirium and related complications. Non-pharmacologic interventions and treatment of the underlying cause/s are the first step of the management. For initial symptom management, non-pharmacological approaches are the first-line strategy and include discontinuation or dose reduction of anticholinergic and psychoactive drugs, family, or companion involvement for reorientation and comfort (Inouye et al. 2014). At this stage, all the risk factors for delirium as shown in Table 5.1 should be eradicated. All these interventions may decrease the incidence of delirium up to 40% (Isik 2014; Kalish et al. 2014; Inouye et al. 1999).

Suicidality, violence potential, fall risk, and wandering risk, inadvertent self-harm risk should all be assessed with appropriate measures taken to ensure safety. Use of restraints should be minimized as they may increase agitation and hence decrease safety (Hoffmann and Schneider 2007). Detailed medication history should be questioned. The patient should be stabilized in a quiet room if possible. Provision of clocks, calendars, and sunlight from the window are helpful to orientate patients. Early mobilization programs should be applied to patients with limited mobility. Visual and hearing aids should be given to these impairments. Finally, prompt pain management should be supplied to patients (Van Rompaey et al. 2012; Schweickert et al. 2009; Devlin et al. 2012). Initially finger-stick glucose should be obtained. To prevent Wernicke's encephalopathy, 100 mg of intravenous (i.v.) thiamine should always be administered before giving glucose 50 ml of D50W i.v.

Initial screening test for detecting etiology of delirium should include blood workup, including complete blood count, glucose, electrolytes, renal and hepatic tests, thyroid function, cultures, chest x-ray, and urinalysis. Further investigations based on clues from history, physical examination, and previous results are indicated if initial analyses fail (Inouye 1998). Neuroimaging should be done unless there is no obvious cause on the first examination.

*Pharmacologic interventions*: Antipsychotics have been the medication of choice in the treatment of delirium. However, there are no Food and Drug Administration (FDA)-approved medications for delirium, and clinicians must be aware that these drugs for the treatment of delirium can have significant side effects. Thus, the drug should be given in the lowest possible dose for the shortest duration. Also, pharmacologic agents should be reserved for patients with severe agitation, which may result in the interruption of essential medical therapies (e.g., intubation, intra-aortic balloon pumps, dialysis catheters) or which may endanger the safety of the patient, other patients, or staff (Inouye et al. 2014; Inouye 2006; Hoffmann and Schneider 2007).

Haloperidol is considered to be the first choice agent for the pharmacological management of delirium, with its high potency and minimal anticholinergic and cardiovascular side effects. It is recommended to start haloperidol with a dose of 1.0 mg orally or parenterally and to repeat the dose every 20–30 min until the patient is calm enough to participate in the management. Vital signs should be checked before repeating each dose. Subsequently, a maintenance dose of one half of the loading dose should be administered in divided doses over the next 24 h, with tapering doses over the next few days (Inouye 1998; Rana and Morren 2013; Kennedy 2003).

Regarding the newer antipsychotic medications in the treatment of delirium, it was demonstrated that risperidone, olanzapine, and quetiapine were as effective and safe as haloperidol (Yoon et al. 2013). In addition, it was reported that olanzapine might reduce the incidence but increase the duration and severity of delirium (Larsen et al. 2010). Besides these reports, it is essential to keep in mind that these atypical antipsychotic drugs were issued a black box warning by FDA due to their 1.6–1.7 times higher death rate when compared to placebo in patients with dementia (Hoffmann and Schneider 2007).

There are some drugs for the treatment of delirium, which are recommended in certain conditions. Benzodiazepines are used in the cases of withdrawal syndromes from alcohol and sedative–hypnotic drugs, agitation with regard to neuroleptic malignant syndrome, and patients with catatonia or severe extrapyramidal reactions. Lorazepam is the first choice with a starting dose of 0.5–1.0 mg in geriatric population. It does not have active metabolites and has advantages such as its parenteral form and relatively less half-life which is approximately 10–15 h (Rana and Morren 2013; Vardi and Harrington 2014).

Prevention and treatment of delirium in the ICU is very crucial, and studies are generally based on targeting decreasing the opioid requirements, aiming to lower the incidence of delirium. Recently, a new agent with its sedative, analgesic, and anxiolytic properties has revealed satisfactory outcomes. Dexmedetomidine, a centrally acting alpha-2 agonist, is highly selective and has been found to have mild cholinergic activity and to be effective without causing significant respiratory depression unlike other studied medications. However, it is reported to cause bradycardia and hypotension at high infusion rates (Pandharipande et al. 2007; Shehabi et al. 2009; Maldonado 2008).

A few trials have addressed the potential utility of cholinesterase inhibitors for the prevention of postoperative delirium because of the central cholinergic deficiency hypothesis in delirium. But, the results have been disappointing (Hempenius et al. 2011). Melatonin plays a central role in the regulation of the sleep–wake cycle which is frequently disrupted in delirium. In addition, alterations of melatonin metabolism may be effective in development delirium. According to a study, melatonin (5 mg two times before intervention) was reported to be a successful therapeutic agent against postoperative delirium in elderly patient (Sultan 2010). It was demonstrated that 0.5 mg/day of melatonin for up to 14 days was associated with lower delirium risk compared with placebo, and it was recommended that nightly melatonin could have potential protective effect for delirium in elderly patient (Al-Aama et al. 2011). Ramelteon, a melatonin agonist, was found to be associated with a lower risk of delirium (3 vs. 32%) when administered nightly to elderly patients admitted for acute care (Hatta et al. 2014).

In a pilot study, gabapentin reduced the incidence of postoperative delirium. It is not known which mechanism it acts on, perhaps it is effective by reducing pain and opioid administration (Leung et al. 2006).

## 5.5 Prognosis

Delirium has been previously considered to be a transient, reversible condition; however, recent studies (Williams-Russo et al. 1992; Brannstron et al. 1998) have documented that delirium may be more persistent than previously believed. Delirium has deleterious effects on long-term cognitive functioning in elderly patients with dementia. The duration, severity, and underlying cause(s) of delirium may be important in these deleterious effects. It has been documented that at least some patients never recover their baseline level of cognitive functioning. In the emergency departments, delirium causes not only increment in stay of length and health-care cost but also duration of delirium negatively affect 6 months functionality and cognitive performance (Han et al. 2017). The mortality rate of patients with delirium is high and can be as much as 30%. Only one third of patients recover from delirium, with the remaining patients suffering a permanent decline in cognitive function (Siddiqi et al. 2006; Inouye 2006).

**Conclusion**

Delirium is a highly varied syndrome ranging from hypoactive to hyperactive states, with a number of recognized precipitating factors and predisposing factors. It is always a geriatric medical emergency, as it may reflect an underlying acute medical issue, and it may portend or possibly cause worse cognitive and other health outcomes. Therefore, delirium should be recognized properly, and necessary precautions and treatment should be done. Delirium management requires an efficient and accurate diagnostic process and rapid and effective treatment. Given the fact that delirium can be prevented in at least one third of cases, delirium prevention is of special importance.

## References

Al-Aama T, Brymer C, Gutmanis I et al (2011) Melatonin decreases delirium in elderly patients: a randomized, placebo-controlled trial. Int J Geriatr Psychiatry 26:687–694

American Psychiatric Association (2013) Diagnostic and statistical manual, 5th edn. APA Press, Washington, DC

Ansaloni L, Catena F, Chattat R et al (2010) Risk factors and incidence of postoperative delirium in elderly patients after elective and emergency surgery. Br J Surg 97(2):273–280

Bucht G, Gustafson Y, Sandberg O (1999) Epidemiology of delirium. Dement Geriatr Cogn Disord 10:315–318

Brannstron B, Gustafson Y, Norberg A, Winblad B (1998) ADL performance and dependency on nursing care in patients with hip fractures and acute confusion in a task allocation care system. Scand J Caring Sci 5:3–11

Caraceni A, Grassi L (2011) Deliriumacute confusional states in palliative medicine, 2nd edn. Oxford University Press, Oxford

Davis HJ, Muniz-Terrera G, Keage HAD et al (2017) Association of delirium with cognitive decline in late life: a neuropathologic study of 3 population-based cohort studies. JAMA Psychiat 74:244–251

Devlin JW, Al-Qadhee NS, Skrobik Y (2012) Pharmacologic prevention and treatment of delirium in critically ill and non-critically ill hospitalised patients: a review of data from prospective, randomised studies. Best Pract Res Clin Anaesthesiol 26:289

Ely EW, Inouye SK, Bernard GR et al (2001) Delirium in mechanically ventilated patients: validity and reliability of the confusion assessment method for the intensive care unit (CAM-ICU). JAMA 286:2703

Fong TG, Tulebaev SR, Inouye SK (2009) Delirium in elderly adults: diagnosis, prevention and treatment. Nat Rev Neurol 5:210–220

Gross AL, Jones RN, Habtemariam DA et al (2012) Delirium and long-term cognitive trajectory among persons with dementia. Arch Intern Med 172:1324–1331

Han JH, Zimmerman EE, Cutler N et al (2009) Delirium in older emergency department patients: recognition, risk factors, and psychomotor subtypes. Acad Emerg Med 16:193–200

Hatta K, Kishi Y, Wada K et al (2014) Preventive effects of ramelteon on delirium: a randomized placebo-controlled trial. JAMA Psychiat 71(4):397–403

Hempenius L, van Leeuwen BL, van Asselt DZ et al (2011) Structured analyses of interventions to prevent delirium. Int J Geriatr Psychiatry 26:441–450

Hoffmann M, Schneider D (2007) Practice guidelines for the treatment of patients with delirium. In: Skolnik NS (ed) Essential practice guidelines in primary care current clinical practice. Humana Press, Totowa, NJ, pp 341–349

Inouye SK, Bogardus ST Jr, Charpentier PA et al (1999) A multicomponent intervention to prevent delirium in hospitalized older patients. N Engl J Med 340:669–676

Inouye SK, Charpentier PA (1996) Precipitating factors for Delirium in hospitalized elderly persons. Predictive model and interrelationship with baseline vulnerability. JAMA 275: 852–857

Inouye SK (1998) Delirium in hospitalized older patients. Clin Geriatr Med 14(4):745–765

Inouye SK (2006) Delirium in older adults. N Engl J Med 354:1157–1165

Inouye SK, van Dyck CH, Alessi CA et al (1990) Clarifying confusion: the confusion assessment method. A new method for detection of delirium. Ann Intern Med 113:941–948

Inouye SK, Viscoli CM, Horwitz RI et al (1993) A predictive model for Delirium in hospitalized elderly medical patients based on admission characteristics. Ann Intern Med 119: 474–481
Inouye SK, Westendorp RG, Saczynski JS (2014) Delirium in elderly people. Lancet 383: 911–922
Isik AT (2014) Geriatrik Olgularda Deliryum/Delirium in The Elderly. İzmir Guven Kitap, Turkey, Izmir. ISBN: 978-605-60355
Han JH, Vasilevskis EE, Chandrasekhar R et al (2017) Delirium in the Emergency Department and Its Extension into Hospitalization (DELINEATE) study: effect on 6-month function and cognition. J Am Geriatr Soc 65(6):1333–1338
Kalish VB, Gillham JE, Unwin BK (2014) Delirium in older persons: evaluation and management. Am Fam Physician 90(3):150–158
Kennedy GJ (2003) Dementia. In: Cassel CK, Leipzig RM, Cohen HJ, Larson EB, Meier DE (eds) Geriatric medicine: an evidence based approach, 4th edn. Springer, New York, pp 1079–1093
Larsen KA, Kelly SE, Stern TA et al (2010) Administration of olanzapine to prevent postoperative delirium in elderly joint-replacement patients: a randomized, controlled trial. Psychosomatics 51(5):409–418
Leung JM, Sands LP, Rico M et al (2006) Pilot clinical trial of gabapentin to decrease postoperative delirium in older patients. Neurology 67(7):1251–1253
Maldonado JR (2008) Delirium in the acute care setting: characteristics, diagnosis and treatment. Crit Care Clin 24(4):657–722
Morandi A, Davis D, Fick DM et al (2014) Delirium superimposed on dementia strongly predicts worse outcomes in older rehabilitation inpatients. JAMA 15:349–354
Pandharipande PP, Pun BT, Herr DL et al (2007) Effect of sedation with dexmedetomidine vs lorazepam on acute brain dysfunction in mechanically ventilated patients: the MENDS randomized controlled trial. JAMA 298(22):2644–2653
Rana AQ, Morren JA (2013) Delirium, neurological emergencies in clinical practice. Springer, London, pp 15–23
Richardson SJ, Davis DHJ, Bellelli G et al (2017) Detecting delirium superimposed on dementia: diagnostic accuracy of a simple combined arousal and attention testing procedure. Int Psychogeriatr 31:1–9
Saxena S, Lawley D (2009) Delirium in the elderly: a clinical review. Postgrad Med J 85(1006):405–413
Schweickert WD, Pohlman MC, Pohlman AS et al (2009) Early physical and occupational therapy in mechanically ventilated, critically ill patients: a randomised controlled trial. Lancet 373(9678):1874–1882
Shehabi Y, Grant P, Wolfenden H et al (2009) Prevalence of delirium with dexmedetomidine compared with morphine based therapy after cardiac surgery: a randomized controlled trial (DEXmedetomidine COmpared to Morphine-DEXCOM study). Anesthesiology 111(5):1075–1084
Siddiqi N, House AO, Holmes JD (2006) Occurrence and outcome of delirium in medical inpatients: a systematic literature review. Age Ageing 35:350–364
Soysal P, Kaya D, Isik AT (2015) Current concepts in the diagnosis, pathophysiology, and treatment of delirium: a European perspective. Curr Geri Rep 4:284–289
Sultan SS (2010) Assessment of role of perioperative melatonin in prevention and treatment of postoperative delirium after hip arthroplasty under spinal anesthesia in the elderly. Saudi J Anaesth 4:169–173
Tomlinson EJ, Phillips NM, Mohebbi M, Hutchinson AM (2017) Risk factors for incident delirium in an acute general medical setting: a retrospective case-control study. J Clin Nurs 26(5–6):658–667
Van Rompaey B, Elseviers MM, Van Drom W et al (2012) The effect of earplugs during the night on the onset of delirium and sleep perception: a randomized controlled trial in intensive care patients. Crit Care 16:R73

Vardi K, Harrington CJ (2014) Delirium: treatment and prevention (part 2). R I Med J 97(6): 24–28

Williams-Russo P, Urquhart BL, Sharrock NE, Charlson ME (1992) Postoperative delirium: predictors and prognosis in elderly orthopedic patients. J Am Geriatr Soc 40:759–767

Yoon HJ, Park KM, Choi WJ et al (2013) Efficacy and safety of haloperidol versus atypical antipsychotic medications in the treatment of delirium. BMC Psychiatry 13:240

# 6 The US Geriatric Psychiatry Approach to Delirium

Neil Evans and George T. Grossberg

## 6.1 Introduction

Delirium is a perturbation of the baseline cognitive equilibrium. It can have a wide variety of cognitive effects. It manifests in a decrease of attention, irritability, arousal, mood, amnesia, and disturbed cognition. Every time a patient is admitted to the hospital, they have an age-stratified risk of developing delirium. The hospital experience is jarring and can easily disrupt a patient's circadian rhythm and sense of normality and strains the patient's cognitive reserves. This is especially present in the ICU where often the patient's perception of days and nights merges. Length of hospital stay and days on a ventilator is strongly correlated with delirium. Greater than 50% of patients will have delirium during a prolonged ICU stay (Mattar et al. 2013). Consequences of delirium include doubling of the rate of cognitive decline of dementia. This results in earlier functional disability, increased healthcare costs, decreased quality of life, and an increase in mortality (Fong et al. 2017). Also, without resolution of the delirium, patients are 2.9 times more likely to die at 1 year compared to those who had their delirium resolved (Kiely et al. 2009). Currently, it has not been determined if there is a common underlying

N. Evans
Department of Internal Medicine, Saint Louis University School of Medicine, St. Louis, MO, USA

G.T. Grossberg (✉)
Department of Psychiatry and Behavioral Neuroscience, Saint Louis University School of Medicine, St. Louis, MO, USA

Division of Geriatric Medicine, Dementia, Healthy Aging, St. Louis University School of Medicine, St. Louis, MO, USA

Department of Anatomy and Neurobiology, St. Louis University School of Medicine, St. Louis, MO, USA
e-mail: george.grossberg@health.slu.edu



A.T. Isik, G.T. Grossberg (eds.), *Delirium in Elderly Patients*,
https://doi.org/10.1007/978-3-319-65239-9_6

predisposition to dementia and delirium. Similarly, it is unclear whether dementia itself can be caused by the delirium.

## 6.2 Presentation

Delirium represents a disruption of the cognitive equilibrium. This disruption is a product of a cascade of cognitive and physiological events that ultimately progresses to dementia, frailty, functional decline, increased levels of care, morbidity, and mortality. Delirium is a state of confusion and a disturbance of consciousness. It has an altered cognitive equilibrium and a fluctuating course. There can be changes throughout the day, and the patient can have lucid periods, which may coincide with morning rounds, that hide the diagnosis and make input and reports from other caregivers crucial to the care of patients at risk for developing delirium.

The cardinal sign of delirium is the disturbance of attention. For example, the patient may be distractible to minor stimuli like the flow of foot traffic outside the room but relatively inattentive to conversation with direct caregivers or visitors. These patients have difficulty with competing thoughts; they are unable to maintain a normal stream of consciousness and lack directed thought processes. They are unable to focus on goal-directed behaviors and unable to order symbols or follow sequenced commands or perform sequenced activities like tying a shoe.

The recognition of delirium is frequently delayed because its most early signs are subtle (Young et al. 2010). This prodromal phase includes subtle thinking changes and sleep disturbance that may be more pronounced in the evening. These initial small changes may only be appreciated by a family member.

There is a spectrum of subtypes of delirium: hyperactive, hypoactive, and mixed. For example, some patients present with increased vigilance, others with psychomotor and autonomic overactivity with agitation, and yet others with tremulousness and visual hallucinations. The different presentations may have different pathophysiological combinations that disrupt the cognitive equilibrium (Fong et al. 2009).

Another more insidious presentation is that of hypoactive delirium. This type of delirium is pervasive and likely underdiagnosed (Fong et al. 2009). It may be the most difficult to diagnose because the symptoms may be vague or subtle or confused for depression with severe fatigue (Fong et al. 2009; Kalish et al. 2014). These patients present with confusion, somnolence, and decreased arousal. The frequency of hypoactive delirium increases with age and is the most common presentation of delirium in palliative care and hospice settings (Kalish et al. 2014).

## 6.3 Costs

Delirium is associated with profound healthcare system costs but also costs to the patient. In a 2014 analysis of post-hip fracture surgery patients, the incidence of postoperative delirium was 28.6%, and each day of delirium increased the hazard of dying at 6 months by 17% (Bellelli et al. 2014). In a study of patients who underwent elective surgery with postoperative ICU admission, the 6-month mortality was 32% in patients with hypoactive delirium compared with 8.7% in the other types of delirium (Cavallazzi et al. 2012).

Attempts have been made to quantify the cost burden of delirium to the healthcare system. Healthcare costs for the average patient with delirium are roughly two and half times greater than for a patient without delirium given similar clinical characteristics during a given hospitalization. Per patient, delirium's total cost ranges from $16 to 64 k. Factoring in the prevalence of the disease, delirium costs 38–152 billion USD annually (Leslie et al. 2008). The type of delirium influences its costs, and hypoactive delirium is the costliest. More than a third of the delirious patients have the hypoactive delirium (Bellelli et al. 2016). Early diagnosis and treatment of delirium provides an opportunity for a substantial reduction in healthcare costs and improvements in quality of life.

The time course of the disease is related to its high healthcare cost; delirium was thought to be completely reversible, but sequelae are nearly ubiquitous. If delirium does develop, there is evidence that some older patients do not recover quickly nor at all, and the persistence of delirium is associated with adverse outcomes and need for ongoing high levels of care (Cole et al. 2009; McAvay et al. 2006). Hshieh et al. showed clinically meaningful impairment in postoperative patients who developed delirium for up to 18 months (Hshieh et al. 2017).

The reversibility of delirium depends on the pathophysiological cause. If the cause was medications, electrolyte disturbance, or infection, there is a higher likelihood of reversing an episode of delirium. However, patients are at higher risk of permanent cognitive disruption if their source of delirium was hypoxia or global metabolic encephalopathy. Delirium increases the odds of having dementia by eightfold. Delirium is associated with a loss of 0.4–1 point on mini-mental status exam each year subsequently (Davis et al. 2012, 2017). The rate of cognitive decline after delirium is more rapid with underlying dementia (Davis et al. 2017). Delirium may deplete the cognitive reserves and hasten the rate of cognitive decline.

## 6.4 Incidence

It is important to be vigilant for any cognitive disruption in all patients, but especially those who are at higher risk. Therefore, knowing the general delirium rates among different populations can help guide the allocation of resources for preventing delirium (see Table 6.1). In addition, several risk factors increase the likelihood of a patient having a disrupted cognitive equilibrium. These risks include dementia, age (>65 years), sex (male), frailty, loss of activities of daily living, malnutrition, the use of antipsychotics, feeding tubes, urinary catheters, living in a nursing home, acute pain, renal disease, hepatic disease, emotional distress, other comorbidities, and sleep deprivation (Fong et al. 2009; Leslie et al. 2008; Bellelli et al. 2016; Inouye et al. 2007; Han et al. 2009; Verloo et al. 2016). Also, those who have had a previous episode of delirium are at higher risk of developing delirium (Bush et al. 2014).

**Table 6.1** Delirium rates among different populations

| Patient population | Percentage of patients developing delirium |
|---|---|
| Adult in the community | 1–2 (Fong et al. 2009) |
| General hospital patient | 20 (Kostas et al. 2013; Ryan et al. 2013) |
| General neurology patient | 29 (Bellelli et al. 2016) |
| Recent stroke | 10–48 (Shi et al. 2012) |
| Age < 50 years old | 5 (Ryan et al. 2013) |
| Age > 80 | 35 (Ryan et al. 2013) |
| Vascular dementia | 32 (Hasegawa et al. 2013) |
| Alzheimer's disease | 15 (Hasegawa et al. 2013) |
| Postcardiac surgery unit patients | 26–52 (Brown 2014) |
| Intensive care unit | 70–83 (Pisani et al. 2005) |
| Four weeks after the cancer treatment hematopoietic stem cell transplantation | 50 (Fann et al. 2002) |
| Terminally ill cancer patients | 85 (Breitbart and Alici 2008) |

## 6.5 Pathophysiology

There are multiple proposed pathophysiologic mechanisms for delirium. Specifically, the following hypotheses have been suggested as leading to or coincident with delirium:

- Neurotransmitter alterations
- Neuroinflammatory
- Neuronal aging
- Oxidative stress
- Melatonin and sleep dysregulation

In each patient, cognitive equilibrium disruption may occur due to several processes that may simultaneously lead to dysregulated neuronal activity. Delirium is the ultimate outcome that is caused by dysregulation of neuronal activity secondary to systemic disturbances (Maldonado 2013).

In the 1940s, Engel and Romano showed that delirium was a disturbance of global cortical function. Their seminal work associated delirium with slowing of dominant posterior alpha rhythm and the presence of abnormal slow-wave activity on EEG (Romano and Engel 1944). Delirium-like behavior was observed in patients with alcohol and sedative drug withdrawal; however, these patients predominately demonstrated low-voltage, fast-wave activity (Engel and Romano 1959). Trzepacz in 1989 and 1994 cited subcortical contributions to delirium with brainstem auditory evoked potentials, somatosensory evoked potentials, and neuroimaging studies of the thalamus, basal ganglia, and the pontine reticular formation (Trzepacz et al. 1989; Trzepacz 1994).

## 6.6 Neurotransmitter Mechanisms

Acetylcholine is a well-studied neurotransmitter, and it is implicated in the delirium state. The lack of physiologically active acetylcholine (either by decreased absolute amount or ineffective receptors) has been correlated with the development of delirium. Several studies have used an objective test, the serum anticholinergic activity (SAA) to quantify anticholinergic effects. It has been shown that increased SAA positively correlated with the development of delirium (Mach et al. 1995; Campbell et al. 2009a; Golinger et al. 1987). Measurements of SAA, measured with binding assays with preparations of brain muscarinic receptors, correlate with the severity of delirium in postoperative and medical patients (Mach et al. 1995). In patients with hypoxia and thiamine deficiency, known risk factors for delirium, there is indirect evidence of associated decreased acetylcholine synthesis in the CNS (Mach et al. 1995; Osiezagha et al. 2013; Yogaratnam et al. 2013; Hshieh et al. 2008). It is important to note that while overall decreases in acetylcholine levels have been implicated in the pathophysiology of acetylcholine, increasing acetylcholine levels to baseline is not necessarily correlated with the amelioration of delirium (Hshieh et al. 2008).

Many medications taken by older adults have anticholinergic activity, even if the primary mechanism of drug is not anticholinergic (Chew et al. 2008). Therefore, it is important to consider medication effects in any adult at risk for delirium, as they can contribute to deterioration of the patient's cognitive equilibrium. Other neurotransmitters have also been implicated in the pathophysiology of delirium. Dopamine excess, disturbances in serotonin, and gamma-aminobutyric acid (GABA) are among the neurotransmitters studied in this context (Maclullich et al. 2008; Sapolsky 1996).

## 6.7 Neuroinflammatory and Oxidative Stress Hypotheses

The neuroinflammatory hypothesis, per Cerejeira et al., involves "acute peripheral inflammatory stimulation induces activation of brain parenchymal cells, expression of proinflammatory cytokines, and inflammatory mediators in the central nervous system" (Cerejeira et al. 2010). Cytokine release and other neuroinflammatory mediators decrease perfusion and oxygenation, leading to decreased cerebral oxidative metabolism. There is an increase in the blood-brain barrier (BBB) permeability leading to neuronal and synaptic dysfunction. The hypothesized BBB disruption and the presence of the inflammatory mediators from the systemic inflammation affect microglial cells and activate and modulate nearby cells, leading to the cognitive and behavioral symptoms of delirium (Maldonado 2013; Cerejeira et al. 2010; Butterworth 2013, 2015). There have been correlations of increased inflammatory mediators C-reactive protein, interleukin IL-1 and IL-6 tumor necrosis factors in delirious patients lending support to this hypothesis (Ritchie et al. 2014; Vasilevskis et al. 2012; George and Mukaetova-Ladinska 2007; Sheldon et al. 1993; de Rooij et al. 2007; Murray et al. 2012).

The activated immune system, as discussed above, can contribute to oxidative damage in the brain at the cellular level. Cellular aging, hypoperfusion, and infection all lead to the formation of reactive oxygen species (ROS) (Aliev et al. 2010; He et al. 2010; Gao et al. 2008). Aliev et al. have proposed this damages the blood-brain barrier through leukocyte adhesion to endothelial cells. The endothelial cells, which are the primary component of the blood-brain barrier, suffer impaired barrier function after leukocyte adhesion. This ultimately leads to increased permeability to ROS and thus oxidative stress in the brain (Aliev et al. 2010). The cycle continues as free radicals are implicated in systemic cellular damage and have been shown to further deteriorate the BBB, leading to increased endothelial permeability (Aliev et al. 2010; He et al. 2010; Hala 2007). The increased permeability allows increased fluid shifts into the brain with perivascular edema formation. At the cellular level, increased edema fluid can decrease perfusion and make oxygen diffusion more difficult. This ultimately leads to microcirculatory impairment and possible ischemic injury or dysfunction (Maldonado 2013). To support this theory further, deficiency in the antioxidant vitamin C is a known contributor to age-related cognitive decline and Alzheimer's disease (Harrison 2012). Pursuant to the previous discussion of neurotransmitter function in the pathogenesis of delirium, acetylcholine synthesis may be particularly sensitive hypoxic injury (Hshieh et al. 2008; Hirsch and Gibson 1984; Cinalli et al. 2013).

## 6.8 Neuronal Aging Hypothesis

The neuronal aging hypothesis derives from observations that there is an increased frequency of delirium in patients over 65 (Maldonado 2013; McNicoll et al. 2003). The probability of transitioning to a delirious state after administration of lorazepam increases by 2% per year after age 65 (Pandharipande et al. 2006). As we age, there is an increased vulnerability to stressors because of a lack of physiologic reserve (Troncale 1996). There are multifactorial reasons that include altered levels of neurotransmitters, blood flow to the brain decreases, and neuron loss (Kochunov et al. 2009; Kelly et al. 2006; Juraska and Lowry 2012; Chen et al. 2011). Neuronal aging helps to explain why younger patients frequently can tolerate greater stress conditions than elderly with a gradually decreasing physiologic reserve before the development of delirium (Maldonado 2013). Additionally, the presence of compromised cognitive abilities before a stressful event is associated with an increase in the incidence of delirium in medical and surgical patients (McNicoll et al. 2003; Franco et al. 2010; Litaker et al. 2001).

## 6.9 Melatonin and Sleep Dysregulation Hypothesis

Melatonin and sleep dysregulation hypothesis focuses on the disruption of the usual stages of sleep that occurs in hospitalized or stressed patients. Sleep deprivation itself has been associated with delirium, and this condition is quite prevalent in hospitalized patients (Flannery et al. 2016).

The 24-h circadian cycle is maintained by light exposure and other factors which affects melatonin secretion. Its disruption can lead to delirium (Fong et al. 2017; Bellelli et al. 2016; Hshieh et al. 2017; Davis et al. 2017; Verloo et al. 2016; Flannery et al. 2016; Fitzgerald et al. 2016; Taito et al. 2016a, b; Bellani et al. 2016; Chen et al. 2016; Dubb et al. 2016; Foster et al. 2016; Hodgson et al. 2016; Kuladee and Prachason 2016; Mo et al. 2016; Morris et al. 2016; Moss et al. 2016; Simel and Rennie 2016).

Melatonin has sleep-wake cycle regulatory effects and helps to reset the circadian rhythm if it is disturbed. Studies in the ICU environment have shown improved quality of sleep, and there are suggestions that prophylactic use may decrease the incidence of delirium (Fong et al. 2017; Bellelli et al. 2016; Hshieh et al. 2017; Davis et al. 2017; Verloo et al. 2016; Flannery et al. 2016; Fitzgerald et al. 2016; Taito et al. 2016a, b; Bellani et al. 2016; Chen et al. 2016; Dubb et al. 2016; Foster et al. 2016; Hodgson et al. 2016; Kuladee and Prachason 2016; Mo et al. 2016; Morris et al. 2016; Moss et al. 2016; Simel and Rennie 2016; Bourne et al. 2008; Sultan 2010; de Jonghe et al. 2014).

The multiple hypotheses of delirium complement and overlap with one another. There are multiple possible mechanisms that likely work in concert to produce the disruption of cognitive equilibrium and that clinicians see as the various manifestations of delirium (e.g., hyperactive, mixed, and hypoactive delirium) (Table 6.2).

## 6.10 Diagnosis

The diagnosis of delirium requires multidisciplinary vigilance and a low threshold for diagnosis. In a study by Inouye in 2001, on the sole basis of clinical judgement, nurses diagnosed 19% of patients with delirium (Inouye et al. 2001). To improve detection of delirium, it is important to know which patients are more susceptible to delirium.

In general, the most important risk factors for delirium are advanced age, preexisting cognitive impairment (e.g., major neurocognitive disorders such as Alzheimer's disease, vascular dementia), and multiple prescribed and over-the-counter medication usage (Bush et al. 2014; Hugo and Ganguli 2014).

The key to diagnosing early is identifying cognitive equilibrium changes. Certain patients have an increased probability of developing delirium (Table 6.1). For at-risk patients, multidisciplinary interaction is beneficial, including the patients' visitors, families, nurses, and physicians. Family members often have a better understanding of changes in cognitive equilibrium and may aid in the diagnosis (Inouye et al. 2001). Also helpful are afternoon and nighttime observations as the fluctuating mental status may worsen secondary to circadian processes.

Currently, DSM V (Table 6.3) criteria are used to diagnose delirium. The most accepted, validated, and rapid screening tool is the Confusion Assessment Method (CAM). The test looks for changes in mental status, distractibility, disorganized thinking, and the level of consciousness (e.g., hypervigilance versus somnolence).

**Table 6.2** List of common drugs that can cause delirium

| Prescription drugs | |
|---|---|
| Central acting agents | • Anticholinergics (oxybutynin)<br>• Anticonvulsants (barbiturates)<br>• Antiparkinsonian agents (benztropine, trihexyphenidyl, and selegiline)<br>• Benzodiazepines (the medication and the withdrawal)<br>• Hypnotics (trazodone) |
| Analgesics | • Opiates (especially meperidine)<br>• Nonsteroidal anti-inflammatory drugs (case reports of COX-2 inhibitors)<br>• Ketamine |
| Antihistamines | • First generation (diphenhydramine) |
| Gastrointestinal agents | • Antispasmodics<br>• $H_2$ blockers |
| Antinauseants | • Scopolamine<br>• Dimenhydrinate |
| Antibiotics | • Fluoroquinolones |
| Psychotropic medications | • Tricyclic antidepressants<br>• Lithium |
| Cardiac medications | • Disopyramide<br>• Digitalis<br>• Antihypertensives (β-blockers, methyldopa, and diuretics) |
| Miscellaneous | • Skeletal muscle relaxants<br>• High-dose steroids |
| Over-the-counter medications and complementary/alternative medications | • Tylenol PM, Motrin PM, Aleve PM (the PM component is diphenhydramine, a potent anticholinergic)<br>• Antinauseants (dimenhydrinate, scopolamine)<br>• Mandrake root, jimsonweed, *Atropa belladonna*, and henbane (contain scopolamine and anticholinergic compounds)<br>• Medications combined with alcohol<br>• Alcohol and its withdrawal |

Adapted from: Alagiakrishnan and Wiens (2004)

**Table 6.3** Condensed DSM V delirium criteria

| |
|---|
| An acute change from baseline in attention and orientation |
| With an additional cognitive disturbance (i.e., memory, language, perception, or vision) |
| That is not better explained by an established or evolving neurocognitive disorder |

One of the difficulties with the CAM is the requirement of additional training before being able to perform it correctly. Another screening tool which has promise is the Global Attentiveness Rating (GAR). The test involves a 2-min or longer conversation with the patient performed by the clinician. At the conclusion, the clinician answers the question: "How well did the patient maintain attention with you during the interview?" A score of ten is perfect engagement and zero is no communication.

The history of the present illness needs to be obtained from a reliable informant/caregiver. It is important to ascertain any recent and chronic illnesses, kidney or liver compromise, medication lists, herbs/supplements, over-the-counter medications, how and when they are taken, substance abuse whether drugs or ethanol, recent psychiatric history, and cognitive baseline (Fig. 6.1). These factors will help to understand the patient's baseline cognitive equilibrium.

## 6.11 Head-to-Toe Analysis

After the patient is identified as having delirium, the next step is to identify potentially reversible causes and/or contributors (Fig. 6.1). It begins with a thorough assessment of the history. This is followed by a whole-body assessment (Fig. 6.2). General physical examination is challenging in a confused and agitated patient but is important to pursue to the extent the patient allows. Vital signs with pulse rate, pulse oximetry, temperature, and BP with orthostatic changes (Fig. 6.1). The hydration status of skin and mucus membrane condition, as well as any possible infectious conditions, are important.

The neurologic exam may be challenging due to poor cooperation and inattention in a patient with delirium. Assessment focuses on assessing for changes from the patient's baseline cognitive equilibrium. This includes documenting the patient's level of consciousness and the extent of attentiveness. If possible, cranial nerve exam including visual fields and motor exam are important to rule out focal neurologic etiologies. Indicated diagnostic tests include urinalysis, complete blood count, chest x-ray, complete metabolic panel, thyroid hormone levels, and toxicology screen (Fig. 6.1).

| History | Diagnostic Tests | As Needed |
|---|---|---|
| Medication List | Urinalysis | ABG |
| Over the Counter Medications | Urine Drug Screen | CT Scan |
| Herbs and Supplements | Glucose Levels | MRI |
| Drugs and Alcohol History | Hemoglobin Levels | Lumbar Puncture |
| Psychiatric History | Electrolytes (Ca, Na, Mg, $PO_4$) | Electroencephalogram |
| Current Medical History | Temperature | Vitamin B12 Levels |
| Recurrent Illnesses | Blood Pressure | |
| Trauma | Osmolality | |
| Sleep History | Thyroid Hormone Levels | |
| Bowel and Urinary History | Parathyroid Hormone Levels | |
| Hydration History | Pancreatic Enzymes | |
| Baseline Mental Status and Mobility | Liver and Kidney Function Tests | |
| | Pharmaceutical Drug Levels | |
| | X-ray for Pneumonia | |

**Fig. 6.1** Important information to obtain

**Head to Toe Differential Diagnosis for Possible Causes of Delirium**

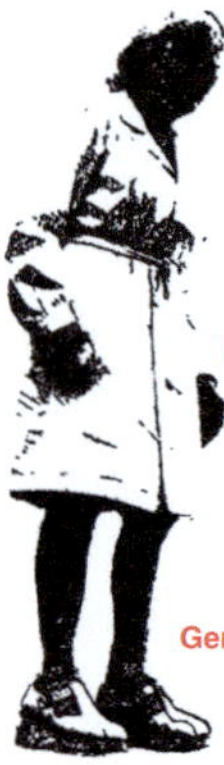

| | |
|---|---|
| Overall | TIA, cerebrovascular accident, subdural hematoma, post-ictal state, trauma, needle track marks, abuse, anemia, chronic pulmonary disease, sepsis, hypothermia, hyperthermia, leukemic blast cell crisis, thrombocytosis, alcohol abuse, malnutrition, sleep deprivation, bipolar, depression, delusions, hallucinations, withdrawal, and Wernicke's Encephalopathy. |
| HEENT | Head: Central nervous system infections, seizures, stroke.<br>Eyes: Decreased visual acuity, acute angle closure glaucoma, retinal artery occlusion, vitreous hemorrhage.<br>Ears: Deafness, presbycusis, ear infection, tinnitus.<br>Nose: Sinus infection, influenza.<br>Throat/Mouth: Cavities, retropharyngeal abscess. |
| Neck/ Hormonal | Thyroid toxicosis, hyperparathyroidism, adrenal insufficiency or overactivity, hyper or hypoglycemia. |
| Chest | Myocardial infarction, angina, coronary artery dissection, bronchitis, pneumonia, pleuritis, pulmonary embolism, asthma exacerbation, aspiration, and shingles. |
| Digestive Tract | Constipation, stool retention, bowel obstruction, peptic ulcer disease, pancreatitis, acute liver failure, cholecystitis, mesenteric ischemia, diverticulitis. |
| Genitourinary Tract | Urinary Retention, urinary tract infection, kidney stone, acute kidney injury, sexual transmitted diseases, hernia, bacterial vaginosis, pelvic prolapse, vulvar irritation, prostatitis, epididymitis. |

**Fig. 6.2** Head-to-toe differential diagnosis for possible causes of delirium

## 6.12 Differential

After a complete but directed history is obtained as described in Fig. 6.1, the causes described in Fig. 6.2 should also be considered, and it is also important to distinguish delirium from nonconvulsive status epilepticus, sundowning, worsening of dementia, and primary psychiatric illnesses. Nonconvulsive status epilepticus may be the most frequently missed diagnosis in the elderly presenting with altered mental status. It can present as a postictal confusion lasting without other signs suggesting status epilepticus, sudden stupor, confusion with hallucinations, and stroke-like symptoms that can disappear. It is a condition that does not have the classic ictal features. It is important if suspected to perform an EEG (Beyenburg et al. 2007). Dementia can have disorientation and difficulty with memory, but changes are frequently more progressive. Dementia with Lewy bodies may also have visual hallucinations like delirium (Scott and Barrett 2007). Sundowning frequently occurs in a patient with dementia, and its symptoms include increased confusion, restlessness, hallucinations, verbal outbursts, and wandering fluctuating loss of attention in a patient. It is important to get a clear cognitive baseline for patients with sundowning and patients with dementia (Evans and Grossberg 2016). Depression can present with reduced concentration symptoms similar to hypoactive delirium but will not fluctuate to the same extent. Assessing the patient at multiple times of the day or asking other caregivers can help rule it out. Mania can appear like delirium with agitation as it can present with attention difficulties, hallucinations, impulsivity, recklessness, and psychotic behavior. The hallucinations in mania will typically be auditory rather than visual and the speech will be pressured. It is important to get a family history and a psychiatric history to help rule it out (Hilty et al. 2006).

## 6.13 Treatment

The best treatment is prevention and the maintenance of vigilance for cognitive equilibrium changes. The early bedside application of the CAM criteria by all staff detects early perturbations in cognitive equilibrium. Close attention will reveal fluctuating mental status, inattention, altered level of consciousness, or disorganized thinking. All these observations may help with early identification of delirium. Combined preventive strategies appear to be effective in preventing delirium (Litaker et al. 2001; Clegg and Young 2011). First, one must identify and reverse the acute cause or causes to the extent that is possible. Early approach includes treating fluid and electrolyte imbalances, improving nutritional status, and treating infections. Modifying risk factors in the environment of the patient is a powerful way to help reduce and ameliorate delirium once it has developed; this includes maintaining supportive care with regular reorientation to person, place, time, and reasons for admission. Measures to reduce anxiety, reassuring family members, and surrounding the patient with familiar objects, visible clocks, and calendars with easily read characters also assist in the treatment of delirium. It is imperative to maintain adequate hydration and feeding and to avoid sleep deprivation by protecting normal sleep cycles. Also, correcting vision and hearing impairment is a priority as the loss of these senses can be very emotionally and cognitively disruptive.

Limiting unnecessary medications and withdrawal from benzodiazepines, barbiturates, selective serotonin reuptake inhibitors, alcohol, and other drugs is useful to remove any potential contributing substances to the delirium (Fong et al. 2009).

It is important to have a low threshold for treatment of pain. Pain medications should be provided on a scheduled basis as patients with delirium may have a difficult time reporting pain. Pain regimens should be centered around non-opioid agents, preferring acetaminophen and lidocaine patches if applicable. If there remain symptoms of pain, consider elevating analgesia with short-acting oral opioids with extreme caution as opioids can worsen delirium (Fong et al. 2006). Prophylactic bowel regimens may prevent and treat possible constipation and urinary retention issues (Manepalli et al. 1990). Monitoring of intake and output will assure that the patient has appropriate hydration and nutrition and will monitor for urinary or fecal retention as these are common causes of delirium (Gower et al. 2012). Ensure the patient is upright when eating to prevent aspiration. Thiamine deficiency is common in the elderly, and alcohol use disorder can be difficult to detect in this population; therefore, thiamine supplementation should be considered. With less evidence, other vitamins may also be considered for supplementation, folate and B12. Encourage a return to baseline activity levels by ambulating out of bed if possible and physical therapy-type activity (Taito et al. 2016b; Robinson and Eiseman 2008).

Disturbances in circadian rhythms have been reported as a potential contributor and effect of delirium. Improving circadian rhythms via good sleep hygiene, e.g., ensuring regular wake times and scheduled bedtimes, is important. It is important to refrain from interrupting these patients with midnight venipuncture, medications, and vital sign checks. There is also emerging evidence that melatonin given prophylactically prevents elderly patients from becoming delirious when presenting to medical wards, though no difference was found when presenting to the surgical wards (Sultan 2010; de Jonghe et al. 2014). Melatonin also has been shown to improve agitated behaviors in delirium (Breitbart and Alici 2012; Al-Aama et al. 2011). One should minimize the use of chemical or physical restraints, as this can worsen or even precipitate delirium (Leslie et al. 2008; Inouye et al. 2007). In patients with agitation/aggressivity and/or psychosis in the context of delirium, short-term use of pharmacotherapy may be indicated.

Table 6.4 reviews various pharmacologic agents which may be useful to prevent harm to self/others or to give time to evaluate for potentially reversible etiologies. Haloperidol is considered the drug of choice for hospital-associated delirium by many healthcare professionals and professional guidelines (Flaherty et al. 2011; Schrijver et al. 2016).

The practice guideline for the treatment of patients with delirium states the first-line agent to treat the hyperactive symptoms of delirium is titrated haloperidol beginning with 0.5 mg (Trzepacz et al. 2010). If extrapyramidal side effects are seen early in the treatment with haloperidol, consider the possibility of Lewy body dementia or Parkinson's disease. If there is an allergy to haloperidol,

**Table 6.4** Pharmacological therapy for delirium

| Drug | Dose | Adverse effects | Comments |
|---|---|---|---|
| *Antipsychotics* | | | |
| Haloperidol | 0.5–1 mg orally or intramuscularly; can repeat every 4 h (orally) or every 60 min (intramuscularly) | Extrapyramidal syndrome, prolonged QT interval, insomnia | Randomized, controlled trials demonstrate reduction in symptom severity and duration |
| *Atypical antipsychotics* | | | |
| Risperidone | 0.5 mg twice daily | Extrapyramidal syndrome, prolonged QT interval, drowsiness<br>Sedation, orthostasis | Randomized, controlled trials comparing efficacy against haloperidol showed comparable response rates |
| Olanzapine | 2.5–5 mg daily | | |
| Quetiapine | 25 mg, 2–3 times daily | | |
| *Benzodiazepines* | | | |
| Lorazepam | 0.5–1 mg orally; can repeat every 4 h | Paradoxical excitation, respiratory depression, excessive sedation, confusion, long acting | Did not show improvement in condition; treatment limited by adverse effects.<br>Benzodiazepines can worsen delirium and should be avoided |
| *Cholinesterase inhibitors* | | | |
| Donepezil | 5 mg daily | Nausea, vomiting, diarrhea, bradycardia | No randomized, controlled studies have been conducted.<br>Not recommended |

Modified from Fong et al. (2009), Candy et al. (2012), and Breitbart et al. (1996)

atypical antipsychotics may also be considered (Schrijver et al. 2016; Trzepacz et al. 2010; Campbell et al. 2009b; Tampi et al. 2015). For further information, see Table 6.4.

**Conclusion**

In the hospital population, disruption to the fragile cognitive equilibrium can result in delirium. It is important to have vigilance with at-risk populations, including elderly, severely ill, and recently operated upon patients. Evaluation should include routine utilization of the CAM as a standard screening device. Preventive care, including prompt evaluation and treatment of precipitating conditions, withdrawal from alcohol and other drugs and medications, frequent reorientations, and good sleep practices, can prevent and may reduce the severity of subsequent delirium. Early diagnosis, evaluation, and treatment of precipitating conditions, combined with aggressive multimodal treatments, can result in a more favorable prognosis in patients with cognitive equilibrium changes and can improve the acute and long-term impact on the patient, family, and caregivers.

## References

Al-Aama T, Brymer C, Gutmanis I, Woolmore-Goodwin SM, Esbaugh J, Dasgupta M (2011) Melatonin decreases delirium in elderly patients: a randomized, placebo-controlled trial. Int J Geriatr Psychiatry 26(7):687–694

Alagiakrishnan K, Wiens CA (2004) An approach to drug induced delirium in the elderly. Postgrad Med J 80(945):388–393

Aliev G, Palacios HH, Gasimov E, Obrenovich ME, Morales L, Leszek J et al (2010) Oxidative stress induced mitochondrial failure and vascular hypoperfusion as a key initiator for the development of alzheimer disease. Pharmaceuticals (Basel) 3(1):158–187

Bellani G, Laffey JG, Pham T, Fan E, Brochard L, Esteban A et al (2016) Epidemiology, patterns of care, and mortality for patients with acute respiratory distress syndrome in intensive care units in 50 countries. JAMA 315(8):788–800

Bellelli G, Mazzola P, Morandi A, Bruni A, Carnevali L, Corsi M et al (2014) Duration of postoperative delirium is an independent predictor of 6-month mortality in older adults after hip fracture. J Am Geriatr Soc 62(7):1335–1340

Bellelli G, Morandi A, Di Santo SG, Mazzone A, Cherubini A, Mossello E et al (2016) "Delirium Day": a nationwide point prevalence study of delirium in older hospitalized patients using an easy standardized diagnostic tool. BMC Med 14(1):106

Beyenburg S, Elger CE, Reuber M (2007) Acute confusion or altered mental state: consider nonconvulsive status epilepticus. Gerontology 53(6):388–396

Bourne RS, Mills GH, Minelli C (2008) Melatonin therapy to improve nocturnal sleep in critically ill patients: encouraging results from a small randomised controlled trial. Crit Care 12(2):R52

Breitbart W, Alici Y (2008) Agitation and delirium at the end of life: "We couldn't manage him". JAMA 300(24):2898–2910, E1

Breitbart W, Alici Y (2012) Evidence-based treatment of delirium in patients with cancer. J Clin Oncol 30(11):1206–1214

Breitbart W, Marotta R, Platt MM, Weisman H, Derevenco M, Grau C et al (1996) A double-blind trial of haloperidol, chlorpromazine, and lorazepam in the treatment of delirium in hospitalized AIDS patients. Am J Psychiatry 153(2):231–237

Brown CH (2014) Delirium in the cardiac surgical ICU. Curr Opin Anaesthesiol 27(2):117–122

Bush SH, Kanji S, Pereira JL, Davis DH, Currow DC, Meagher DJ et al (2014) Treating an established episode of delirium in palliative care: expert opinion and review of the current evidence base with recommendations for future development. J Pain Symptom Manag 48(2):231–248
Butterworth RF (2013) The liver-brain axis in liver failure: neuroinflammation and encephalopathy. Nature reviews. Gastroenterol Hepatol 10(9):522–528
Butterworth RF (2015) Pathogenesis of hepatic encephalopathy and brain edema in acute liver failure. J Clin Exp Hepatol 5(Suppl 1):S96–S103
Campbell N, Boustani M, Limbil T, Ott C, Fox C, Maidment I et al (2009a) The cognitive impact of anticholinergics: a clinical review. Clin Interv Aging 4:225–233
Campbell N, Boustani MA, Ayub A, Fox GC, Munger SL, Ott C et al (2009b) Pharmacological management of delirium in hospitalized adults—a systematic evidence review. J Gen Intern Med 24(7):848–853
Candy B, Jackson KC, Jones L, Leurent B, Tookman A, King M (2012) Drug therapy for delirium in terminally ill adult patients. Cochrane Database Syst Rev 11:CD004770
Cavallazzi R, Saad M, Marik PE (2012) Delirium in the ICU: an overview. Ann Intensive Care 2(1):49
Cerejeira J, Firmino H, Vaz-Serra A, Mukaetova-Ladinska EB (2010) The neuroinflammatory hypothesis of delirium. Acta Neuropathol 119(6):737–754
Chen JJ, Rosas HD, Salat DH (2011) Age-associated reductions in cerebral blood flow are independent from regional atrophy. NeuroImage 55(2):468–478
Chen S, Shi L, Liang F, Xu L, Desislava D, Wu Q et al (2016) Exogenous melatonin for delirium prevention: a meta-analysis of randomized controlled trials. Mol Neurobiol 53(6):4046–4053
Chew ML, Mulsant BH, Pollock BG, Lehman ME, Greenspan A, Mahmoud RA et al (2008) Anticholinergic activity of 107 medications commonly used by older adults. J Am Geriatr Soc 56(7):1333–1341
Cinalli AR, Guarracino JF, Fernandez V, Roquel LI, Losavio AS (2013) Inosine induces presynaptic inhibition of acetylcholine release by activation of A3 adenosine receptors at the mouse neuromuscular junction. Br J Pharmacol 169(8):1810–1823
Clegg A, Young JB (2011) Which medications to avoid in people at risk of delirium: a systematic review. Age Ageing 40(1):23–29
Cole MG, Ciampi A, Belzile E, Zhong L (2009) Persistent delirium in older hospital patients: a systematic review of frequency and prognosis. Age Ageing 38(1):19–26
Davis DH, Muniz Terrera G, Keage H, Rahkonen T, Oinas M, Matthews FE et al (2012) Delirium is a strong risk factor for dementia in the oldest-old: a population-based cohort study. Brain 135(Pt 9):2809–2816
Davis DH, Muniz-Terrera G, Keage HA, Stephan BC, Fleming J, Ince PG et al (2017) Association of delirium with cognitive decline in late life: a neuropathologic study of 3 population-based cohort studies. JAMA Psychiat 74(3):244–251
Dubb R, Nydahl P, Hermes C, Schwabbauer N, Toonstra A, Parker AM et al (2016) Barriers and strategies for early mobilization of patients in intensive care units. Ann Am Thorac Soc 13(5):724–730
Engel GL, Romano J (1959) Delirium, a syndrome of cerebral insufficiency. J Chronic Dis 9(3):260–277
Evans NR, Grossberg GT (2016) Sundowning: phenomenology, pathophysiology, and treatment approaches. Psychiatry Advisor [Internet]. http://www.psychiatryadvisor.com/alzheimers-disease-and-dementia/sundowning-phenomenology-pathophysiology-and-treatment-approaches/article/524142/. Accessed 17 May 2017
Fann JR, Roth-Roemer S, Burington BE, Katon WJ, Syrjala KL (2002) Delirium in patients undergoing hematopoietic stem cell transplantation. Cancer 95(9):1971–1981
Fitzgerald J, O'Regan N, Adamis D, Timmons S, Dunne C, Trzepacz P, Meagher D (2016) Concordance between the delirium motor subtyping scale (DMSS) and the abbreviated version (DMSS-4) over longitudinal assessment in elderly medical inpatients. Int Psychogeriatr 28:845–851

Flaherty JH, Gonzales JP, Dong B (2011) Antipsychotics in the treatment of delirium in older hospitalized adults: a systematic review. J Am Geriatr Soc 59(Suppl 2):S269–S276

Flannery AH, Oyler DR, Weinhouse GL (2016) The impact of interventions to improve sleep on delirium in the ICU: a systematic review and research framework. Crit Care Med 44(12):2231–2240

Fong HK, Sands LP, Leung JM (2006) The role of postoperative analgesia in delirium and cognitive decline in elderly patients: a systematic review. Anesth Analg 102(4):1255–1266

Fong TG, Tulebaev SR, Inouye SK (2009) Delirium in elderly adults: diagnosis, prevention and treatment. Nat Rev Neurol 5(4):210–220

Fong TG, Inouye SK, Jones RN (2017) Delirium, dementia, and decline. JAMA Psychiat 74(3):212–213

Foster J, Burry LD, Thabane L, Choong K, Menon K, Duffett M et al (2016) Melatonin and melatonin agonists to prevent and treat delirium in critical illness: a systematic review protocol. Syst Rev 5(1):199

Franco JG, Valencia C, Bernal C, Ocampo MV, Trzepacz PT, Pablo J et al (2010) Relationship between cognitive status at admission and incident delirium in older medical inpatients. J Neuropsychiatry Clin Neurosci 22(3):329–337

Gao L, Laude K, Cai H (2008) Mitochondrial pathophysiology, reactive oxygen species, and cardiovascular diseases. Vet Clin North Am Small Anim Pract 38(1):137–155, vi

George J, Mukaetova-Ladinska EB (2007) Delirium and C-reactive protein. Age Ageing 36(2):115–116

Golinger RC, Peet T, Tune LE (1987) Association of elevated plasma anticholinergic activity with delirium in surgical patients. Am J Psychiatry 144(9):1218–1220

Gower LE, Gatewood MO, Kang CS (2012) Emergency department management of delirium in the elderly. West J Emerg Med 13(2):194–201

Hala M (2007) Pathophysiology of postoperative delirium: systemic inflammation as a response to surgical trauma causes diffuse microcirculatory impairment. Med Hypotheses 68(1): 194–196

Han JH, Morandi A, Ely EW, Callison C, Zhou C, Storrow AB et al (2009) Delirium in the nursing home patients seen in the emergency department. J Am Geriatr Soc 57(5):889–894

Harrison FE (2012) A critical review of vitamin C for the prevention of age-related cognitive decline and Alzheimer's disease. J Alzheimers Dis 29(4):711–726

Hasegawa N, Hashimoto M, Yuuki S, Honda K, Yatabe Y, Araki K et al (2013) Prevalence of delirium among outpatients with dementia. Int Psychogeriatr 25(11):1877–1883

He F, Yin F, Peng J, Deng X, Wu L, Zhang C (2010) Molecular mechanism for change in permeability in brain microvascular endothelial cells induced by LPS. Zhong Nan Da Xue Xue Bao Yi Xue Ban 35(11):1129–1137

Hilty DM, Leamon MH, Lim RF, Kelly RH, Hales RE (2006) A review of bipolar disorder in adults. Psychiatry (Edgmont) 3(9):43–55

Hirsch JA, Gibson GE (1984) Selective alteration of neurotransmitter release by low oxygen in vitro. Neurochem Res 9(8):1039–1049

Hodgson CL, Bailey M, Bellomo R, Berney S, Buhr H, Denehy L et al (2016) A binational multicenter pilot feasibility randomized controlled trial of early goal-directed mobilization in the ICU. Crit Care Med 44(6):1145–1152

Hshieh TT, Fong TG, Marcantonio ER, Inouye SK (2008) Cholinergic deficiency hypothesis in delirium: a synthesis of current evidence. J Gerontol A Biol Sci Med Sci 63(7):764–772

Hshieh TT, Saczynski J, Gou RY, Marcantonio E, Jones RN, Schmitt E et al (2017) Trajectory of functional recovery after postoperative delirium in elective surgery. Ann Surg 265(4):647–653

Hugo J, Ganguli M (2014) Dementia and cognitive impairment: epidemiology, diagnosis, and treatment. Clin Geriatr Med 30(3):421–442

Inouye SK, Foreman MD, Mion LC, Katz KH, Cooney LM Jr (2001) Nurses' recognition of delirium and its symptoms: comparison of nurse and researcher ratings. Arch Intern Med 161(20):2467–2473

Inouye SK, Zhang Y, Jones RN, Kiely DK, Yang F, Marcantonio ER (2007) Risk factors for delirium at discharge: development and validation of a predictive model. Arch Intern Med 167(13):1406–1413

de Jonghe A, van Munster BC, Goslings JC, Kloen P, van Rees C, Wolvius R et al (2014) Effect of melatonin on incidence of delirium among patients with hip fracture: a multicentre, double-blind randomized controlled trial. CMAJ 186(14):E547–E556

Juraska JM, Lowry NC (2012) Neuroanatomical changes associated with cognitive aging. Curr Top Behav Neurosci 10:137–162

Kalish VB, Gillham JE, Unwin BK (2014) Delirium in older persons: evaluation and management. Am Fam Physician 90(3):150–158

Kelly KM, Nadon NL, Morrison JH, Thibault O, Barnes CA, Blalock EM (2006) The neurobiology of aging. Epilepsy Res 68(Suppl 1):S5–20

Kiely DK, Marcantonio ER, Inouye SK, Shaffer ML, Bergmann MA, Yang FM et al (2009) Persistent delirium predicts greater mortality. J Am Geriatr Soc 57(1):55–61

Kochunov P, Ramage AE, Lancaster JL, Robin DA, Narayana S, Coyle T et al (2009) Loss of cerebral white matter structural integrity tracks the gray matter metabolic decline in normal aging. NeuroImage 45(1):17–28

Kostas TR, Zimmerman KM, Rudolph JL (2013) Improving delirium care: prevention, monitoring, and assessment. Neurohospitalist 3(4):194–202

Kuladee S, Prachason T (2016) Development and validation of the Thai version of the 4 'A's test for delirium screening in hospitalized elderly patients with acute medical illnesses. Neuropsychiatr Dis Treat 12:437–443

Leslie DL, Marcantonio ER, Zhang Y, Leo-Summers L, Inouye SK (2008) One-year health care costs associated with delirium in the elderly population. Arch Intern Med 168(1):27–32

Litaker D, Locala J, Franco K, Bronson DL, Tannous Z (2001) Preoperative risk factors for post-operative delirium. Gen Hosp Psychiatry 23(2):84–89

Mach JR Jr, Dysken MW, Kuskowski M, Richelson E, Holden L, Jilk KM (1995) Serum anticholinergic activity in hospitalized older persons with delirium: a preliminary study. J Am Geriatr Soc 43(5):491–495

Maclullich AM, Ferguson KJ, Miller T, de Rooij SE, Cunningham C (2008) Unravelling the pathophysiology of delirium: a focus on the role of aberrant stress responses. J Psychosom Res 65(3):229–238

Maldonado JR (2013) Neuropathogenesis of delirium: review of current etiologic theories and common pathways. Am J Geriatr Psychiatry 21(12):1190–1222

Manepalli J, Grossberg GT, Mueller C (1990) Prevalence of delirium and urinary tract infection in a psychogeriatric unit. J Geriatr Psychiatry Neurol 3(4):198–202

Mattar I, Chan MF, Childs C (2013) Risk factors for acute delirium in critically ill adult patients: a systematic review. ISRN Crit Care 2013:1–10

McAvay GJ, Van Ness PH, Bogardus ST Jr, Zhang Y, Leslie DL, Leo-Summers LS et al (2006) Older adults discharged from the hospital with delirium: 1-year outcomes. J Am Geriatr Soc 54(8):1245–1250

McNicoll L, Pisani MA, Zhang Y, Ely EW, Siegel MD, Inouye SK (2003) Delirium in the intensive care unit: occurrence and clinical course in older patients. J Am Geriatr Soc 51(5): 591–598

Mo Y, Scheer CE, Abdallah GT (2016) Emerging role of melatonin and melatonin receptor agonists in sleep and delirium in intensive care unit patients. J Intensive Care Med 31(7): 451–455

Morris PE, Berry MJ, Files DC, Thompson JC, Hauser J, Flores L et al (2016) Standardized rehabilitation and hospital length of stay among patients with acute respiratory failure: a randomized clinical trial. JAMA 315(24):2694–2702

Moss M, Nordon-Craft A, Malone D, Van Pelt D, Frankel SK, Warner ML et al (2016) A randomized trial of an intensive physical therapy program for patients with acute respiratory failure. Am J Respir Crit Care Med 193(10):1101–1110

Murray C, Sanderson DJ, Barkus C, Deacon RM, Rawlins JN, Bannerman DM et al (2012) Systemic inflammation induces acute working memory deficits in the primed brain: relevance for delirium. Neurobiol Aging 33(3):603–616, e3

Osiezagha K, Ali S, Freeman C, Barker NC, Jabeen S, Maitra S et al (2013) Thiamine deficiency and delirium. Innov Clin Neurosci 10(4):26–32

Pandharipande P, Shintani A, Peterson J, Pun BT, Wilkinson GR, Dittus RS et al (2006) Lorazepam is an independent risk factor for transitioning to delirium in intensive care unit patients. Anesthesiology 104(1):21–26

Pisani MA, Redlich CA, McNicoll L, Ely EW, Friedkin RJ, Inouye SK (2005) Short-term outcomes in older intensive care unit patients with dementia. Crit Care Med 33(6): 1371–1376

Ritchie CW, Newman TH, Leurent B, Sampson EL (2014) The association between C-reactive protein and delirium in 710 acute elderly hospital admissions. Int Psychogeriatr 26(5): 717–724

Robinson TN, Eiseman B (2008) Postoperative delirium in the elderly: diagnosis and management. Clin Interv Aging 3(2):351–355

Romano J, Engel GL (1944) Electroencephalographic data. Arch Neurol Psychiatr 51(356)

de Rooij SE, van Munster BC, Korevaar JC, Levi M (2007) Cytokines and acute phase response in delirium. J Psychosom Res 62(5):521–525

Ryan DJ, O'Regan NA, Caoimh RO, Clare J, O'Connor M, Leonard M et al (2013) Delirium in an adult acute hospital population: predictors, prevalence and detection. BMJ Open 3(1)

Sapolsky RM (1996) Stress, glucocorticoids, and damage to the nervous system: the current state of confusion. Stress (Amsterdam, Netherlands) 1(1):1–19

Schrijver EJ, de Graaf K, de Vries OJ, Maier AB, Nanayakkara PW (2016) Efficacy and safety of haloperidol for in-hospital delirium prevention and treatment: a systematic review of current evidence. Eur J Intern Med 27:14–23

Scott KR, Barrett AM (2007) Dementia syndromes: evaluation and treatment. Expert Rev Neurother 7(4):407–422

Sheldon J, Riches P, Gooding R, Soni N, Hobbs JR (1993) C-reactive protein and its cytokine mediators in intensive-care patients. Clin Chem 39(1):147–150

Shi Q, Presutti R, Selchen D, Saposnik G (2012) Delirium in acute stroke: a systematic review and meta-analysis. Stroke 43(3):645–649

Simel DL, Rennie D (2016) Delirium. In: The rational clinical examination: evidence-based clinical diagnosis. McGraw-Hill Education, New York, NY

Sultan SS (2010) Assessment of role of perioperative melatonin in prevention and treatment of postoperative delirium after hip arthroplasty under spinal anesthesia in the elderly. Saudi J Anaesth 4(3):169–173

Taito S, Ota K, Shime N (2016a) Is earlier and more intensive physical therapy program better? Am J Respir Crit Care Med 194(8):1032

Taito S, Shime N, Ota K, Yasuda H (2016b) Early mobilization of mechanically ventilated patients in the intensive care unit. J Intensive Care 4(1):50

Tampi RR, Tampi DJ, Barua S et al (2015) Management of delirium in the elderly patients: a review of evidence. J Drug Abuse 1:1

Troncale JA (1996) The aging process. Physiologic changes and pharmacologic implications. Postgrad Med 99(5):111–114, 20–2

Trzepacz PT (1994) The neuropathogenesis of delirium. A need to focus our research. Psychosomatics 35(4):374–391

Trzepacz PT, Sclabassi RJ, Van Thiel DH (1989) Delirium: a subcortical phenomenon? J Neuropsychiatry Clin Neurosci 1(3):283–290

Trzepacz PT, Breitbart W, Franklin J, Levenson J, Richard Martini D, Wang P (2010) Treatment of patients with delirium. In: Practice Guideline for the treatment of patients with delirium. Trzepacz PT, cheir. American Psychiatric Association, APA Press. 2010

Vasilevskis EE, Han JH, Hughes CG, Ely EW (2012) Epidemiology and risk factors for delirium across hospital settings. Best Pract Res Clin Anaesthesiol 26(3):277–287

Verloo H, Goulet C, Morin D, von Gunten A (2016) Association between frailty and delirium in older adult patients discharged from hospital. Clin Interv Aging 11:55–63
Yogaratnam J, Jacob R, Naik S, Magadi H, Sim K (2013) Prolonged delirium secondary to hypoxic-ischemic encephalopathy following cardiac arrest. Clin Psychopharmacol Neurosci 11(1):39–42
Young J, Murthy L, Westby M, Akunne A, O'Mahony R, Guideline Development G (2010) Diagnosis, prevention, and management of delirium: summary of NICE guidance. BMJ 341:c3704

# 7 Approach to the Elderly Patient with Delirium: A Neurologist's Perspective

Gülsen Babacan-Yildiz

Delirium is a clinical syndrome characterized by acute or subacute disturbances in cognitive functions, wakefulness, diurnal rhythm, motor activities, or perception that are associated with fluctuating psychotic features (Lipowski 1990). For patients with already existing cognitive dysfunction or dementia, a worsening in the previous state of cognition is required to qualify for a diagnosis of delirium.

Delirium, which literally means "*off the track*" in Latin, is frequently described as a state of confusion, and it was originally described as a "*cerebral deficiency syndrome*" by Engel and Romano in 1959. Although there are more than 60 synonyms reported in the literature for delirium, the term "*acute confusional state*" is the most frequently preferred one in the daily clinical practice (Engel and Romano 2004).

## 7.1 Types of Delirium

Delirium is divided into three groups according to the alertness and motor activity:

*Hyperactive delirium*: characterized by increased motor activity and agitated behavior

*Hypoactive delirium*: characterized by decreased motor activity and lethargy

*Mixed-type delirium*: characterized by fluctuations of hypoactive/hyperactive delirium symptoms

Hypoactive and hyperactive delirium states may also exhibit a certain degree of variation in terms of the underlying conditions, the affected areas of the brain, and pathophysiological processes involved. For instance, while withdrawal from benzodiazepines or alcohol is associated with hyperactive delirium, conditions such

G. Babacan-Yildiz, M.D.
Department of Neurology, Medical Faculty, Bezmi Alem Vakıf University,
Adnan Menderes Bulvarı, 34093 Fatih/Istanbul, Turkey
e-mail: gbabacan@hotmail.com



A.T. Isik, G.T. Grossberg (eds.), *Delirium in Elderly Patients*,
https://doi.org/10.1007/978-3-319-65239-9_7

as encephalopathy and benzodiazepine toxicity lead to the development of hypoactive delirium. Also, hyperactive delirium is associated with decreased GABA system activity, increased cerebral metabolism, and increased EEG activity, while overstimulation of the GABA system, decreased global cerebral metabolism, and diffuse slowing down in electroencephalography (EEG) are characteristics for hypoactive delirium (Breitbart and Cohen 2000). Besides, orbitofrontal cortex, cingulate gyrus, and hippocampus are usually affected in patients with hyperactive delirium, while hypoactive delirium generally involves left hemispheric lesions (Trzepacz 2000).

The most frequent type of delirium is the mixed type with an incidence of 42%, followed by hyperactive (30%) and hypoactive (26%) delirium (Inao et al. 2001; Meagher et al. 2000). However, these figures are somewhat different in patients admitted to the intensive care unit (ICU) in whom the mixed type (64%) represents even a higher proportion of patient, followed by hypoactive delirium (35%) and pure hyperactive delirium.

## 7.2 Epidemiology

Delirium incidence increases markedly with age. The prevalence is 0.4%, 1.1%, and 13.6% in individuals >18, >55, or >85 years of age, respectively. In surgical patients, and particularly in those undergoing cardiothoracic, emergency orthopedic, or cataract surgery or in those admitted to the ICU, the incidence is significantly higher (Milstein et al. 2001). Of the adult patients treated in an inpatient facility, 10–20% develop delirium, while this figure is increased to 30–40% among geriatric patients and to 80% in those admitted to an ICU (Ely et al. 2004).

## 7.3 Diagnosis

Delirium is defined in DSM-IV-TR (*Diagnostic and Statistical Manual of Mental Disorders, Fourth Edition, Text Revision*) as a cognitive disorder. So, clinical deterioration in cognitive function is essential for diagnosis. There are 4 basic principles in the DSM-IV-TR criteria for delirium diagnosis: a) disturbance of consciousness (i.e., reduced clarity of awareness of the environment) with reduced ability to focus, sustain or shift attention, b) a change in cognition or the development of a perceptual disturbance that is not better accounted for by a preexisting, established or evolving dementia (hallucitation), c) the disturbance develops over a short period of time (usually hours to days) and tends to fluctuate during the course of the day, d) there is evidence from the history, physical examination or laboratory findings that the disturbance is caused by the direct physiological consequences of a general medical condition (Hales and Yudofsky 2003). Although many scales have been developed to assess delirium symptoms, most of these are not very specific leading to diagnostic difficulties (Schuurmans et al. 2003). One of the most widely used is the MMSE test. However, it is not specific to delirium (Cole et al. 2002). Confusion

Assessment Method (CAM) and CAM-ICU represent standardized scales used for this purpose that assess ten different domains: acute onset and fluctuating course, attention deficit, disorganized thinking and consciousness, orientation and cognitive disorders, memory impairment, psychomotor retardation or agitation, and disturbance in sleep-wake rhythm (Inouye et al. 1990). In a short form of CAM, some domains (acute onset and fluctuating course, attention deficit, disorganized thinking and consciousness) are evaluated. Additionally, Delirium Rating Scale (DRS) and its newer version, DRS-R-98, may also be used to assess delirium. DRS-R-98 is more specific than the original DRS to assess the severity of delirium. Also, DRS-R-98 is the only validated scale on the validity and reliability of evaluating delirium (Trzepacz et al. 2001).

Since the first description of delirium, the diffuse slowing down in the basal EEG activity in patients with delirium is a well-known phenomenon, and serial EEG recordings have been proposed as a useful method for diagnosing delirium (Jacobson and Jerrier 2000). However, until now no consensus has been reached regarding the appropriate EEG electrodes for delirium and the EEG findings that are more specific for delirium. Also the nature of the association between the fluctuating course of delirium and the changes in EEG findings has not been fully elucidated. Due to this fluctuating clinical course, it is imperative that EEG recordings are performed just before or after a diagnosis of delirium, and a prolonged interval between the diagnosis of delirium and EEG recordings increases the risk of misdiagnosis.

Another important issue is represented by the fact that diffuse slowing down of the basal activity in EEG may also be seen in dementia and during sleep, in addition to delirium. However, due to the presence of K-complexes and sleep spindles during sleep, EEG and continuous nature of the diffuse slowing down of basal EEG activity in patients with dementia are characteristics that may assist in the differential diagnosis (Rechtschaffen and Kales 1968). But, despite the specificity of the EEG that is quite high, the sensitivity is lower.

Although an examination of the cerebrospinal fluid (CSF) generally presents practical challenges in patients with delirium, it bears clinical significance in terms of identification of the underlying pathology and in terms of initiating the specific treatments in conditions such as encephalopathy or central nervous system (CNS) infection. Furthermore, measurement of Aβ1–42, tau, and phosphorylated tau in CSF is important for the differential diagnosis of dementia and delirium. On the other hand, delirium developing on the background of dementia complicates this differentiation.

## 7.4 Causes

Possible causes of delirium can be divided into eight categories: induced by drugs, infections, fluid-electrolyte or metabolic imbalances, cranial operations, low perfusion, alcohol and drug withdrawal, and sensory and environmental causes. Risk factors for delirium are generally divided into three groups as predisposing factors, precipitating factors, and facilitating conditions. The most important factor is CNS involvements (Ely et al. 2004).

## 7.5 Pathophysiology

Although delirium in geriatric population is a frequent problem, especially in hospitalized patients, its pathophysiology has not been precisely defined. Despite many potential precipitating factors including neurological conditions such as stroke, dementia, and encephalopathy, delirium may accompany almost all diseases with a generally very similar clinical picture. This suggests the presence of a common pathway and a similar mechanism—probably via multiple pathogenic mechanisms—through which all these factors contribute to the pathophysiology of delirium. It is widely accepted that decreased muscarinic cholinergic activity represents the main neurochemical pathology in delirium and that there is an increased risk of delirium due to the use of medications affecting the activity of acetylcholine (Flacker et al. 1998; Thomas et al. 2008). Cholinergic system plays an important role in cognitive functions such as learning, memory, and attention, and the medial thalamic diffuse projection plays an important role in wakefulness. The simultaneous stimulation of both of these systems results in an imbalance in cholinergic and noradrenergic mechanisms, leading to a combination of cortical inhibition and excitation, corresponding to clinical delirium, characterized by behavioral symptoms.

On the other hand, in addition to acetylcholine, many other neurotransmitters such as dopamine and glutamate as well as melatonin levels are thought to be involved in the brains of delirium patients (Cole 2004; Broadhurst and Wilson 2001; Sharon and Inouye 2006). However, the specific role of these neurotransmitters at different levels and stages of the condition is not fully understood (Caeiro et al. 2004).

Although the primary brain areas involved in patients with delirium are not well known, frontal and temporal lesions play a significant role in hippocampal dysfunction. Also, a recent study found hypoperfusion in frontal and parietal areas as well as in the pons using single-photon emission computed tomography (SPECT) (Fong et al. 2006). Additionally, hypercortisolism resulting from the disturbances in the pituitary-hypophyseal-adrenal axis may play a role in the pathophysiology of delirium, as well as the role of the production of certain cytokines, disturbances in the blood-brain barrier, and oxidative stress (Gustafson et al. 1991). Consequently clinically delirium becomes manifested due to a global impact due to the changes in cellular glucose and oxygen utilization, cellular repair processes, and axonal transport (Maldonado 2008).

## 7.6 Treatment

A multifactorial approach is necessary in the treatment of delirium, since generally there is an underlying condition, and since it may present with a highly heterogeneous clinical picture. Thus, determination of the underlying cause of delirium should be the first step. Therapeutic strategies will be either delayed or inadequate, unless the etiological factors are targeted. On the other hand, although more than one third of the cases with delirium are actually preventable, the heterogeneous nature of the symptoms frequently leads to a delay in diagnosis with a subsequent delay in treatment (Inouye et al. 1999).

To organize environmental factors, to ensure adequate nutrient intake, and to protect the patient from dehydration and constipation are very important. Also to avoid certain drugs, including anticholinergic effects, such as amitriptyline, clindamycin, dexamethasone, phenobarbital, atropine, oxybutynin, digoxin, diltiazem, furosemide, and drugs with codeine, has a very important place in treatment.

Although there is no FDA-approved pharmaceutical agent for the treatment of delirium and the absence of a consensus regarding the definitive evidence for the benefit of commonly used medications, there is a general agreement among the clinicians to initiate medical treatment. It is recommended that the pharmacological therapy be administered in line with the recommendations set out in the American Psychiatric Association (APA) Clinical Practice Guidelines (APA 2000). The most commonly used agent for the treatment of dementia is haloperidol owing to its low potential for anticholinergic side effects, small number of active metabolites, and low potential for sedation and hypotension. Newer antipsychotics such as risperidone or olanzapine may represent safer alternatives than haloperidol, although the experience with these agents is still limited, and even more importantly, both of these agents are associated with an increased risk of stroke (Street et al. 2000; De Deyn et al. 1999; Brodaty et al. 2003). On the other hand, in patients with Parkinsonism, lorazepam may be the agent of choice.

## 7.7 Genetic

There is a relative scarcity of published data on the genetics of delirium, with only one study reporting an association between the apolipoprotein ε4 allele and delirium (Van Munster et al. 2009). The increased risk of delirium in APOEε4 allele carriers may be explained on the basis of the inadequacy of the acetylcholinergic pathway caused by cytokines as shown in animal studies and also on the basis of decreased brain cholinergic activity due to the presence of APOEε4 genotype (Allen et al. 1997).

## 7.8 Delirium in Neurologic Disorders

### 7.8.1 Delirium in Stroke

Stroke is a common neurological syndrome developing due to an acute vascular disorder, and stroke patients represent the most common patient group attending neurology clinics. Although the risk of delirium in stroke patients is already high due to the concomitant predisposing or precipitating risk factors, stroke alone is a risk factor for delirium (Young and Inouye 2007).

Although studies examining patients with delirium developing after stroke are scarce in number, the existing reports suggest a wide risk range for developing delirium, i.e., between 13 and 48%, following ischemic or hemorrhagic stroke. The variability between the reported figures is thought to arise from the differences in patient selection criteria and in the definition of delirium. Approximately 1% of patients with subarachnoid hemorrhage (SAC) may present with delirium. Stroke directly presenting with delirium is a very rare condition (Gustafson et al. 1993; Henon et al. 1999).

Although delirium is a common complication of stroke, the pathophysiological mechanisms responsible for its development have not been accurately or definitively delineated. However, the pathophysiological factors mentioned above also pertain to delirium developing in stroke patients, as with other cases of delirium. A comparison of the risk of delirium following acute coronary syndrome or stroke (13% vs. 2%) demonstrates that brain damage plays a significant role in the pathogenesis of delirium (Caeiro et al. 2004).

The most important independent risk factors for delirium in stroke patients include a deterioration of cognitive functions or dementia preceding the stroke (Langhorne et al. 2000). Although a diagnosis of dementia has already been established and treatment has been initiated in some patients with dementia, in others, the symptoms of dementia may be overlooked due to the insidious course of the condition, leading to a markedly more rapid clinical course together with the occurrence of stroke. Although majority of the studies point out to the advanced age as a risk factor for poststroke delirium, some others claimed that age alone is not a risk factor for the delirium (Sheng et al. 2006). Some authors even reported an association between low educational level and poststroke delirium. Despite the uncertainty surrounding the contribution of the site of the stroke to the risk of delirium, a higher incidence of delirium has been reported in left-sided lesions than those in the contralateral side. In the temporal lobe, fusiform and lingual gyrus, caudate nucleus, and anterior cingulum infarction, acute hyperactive delirium may occur similar to delirium which develops due to alcohol withdrawal (Oldenbeuving et al. 2011).

Most of the patients experiencing a stroke are hospitalized for diagnosis and treatment. However, patients who develop delirium during the inpatient care tend to have prolonged hospital stay, are more likely to require nursing home care and to lose their independence following discharge, and have an increased risk of dementia (Siddiq et al. 2006).

Early recognition and treatment of delirium in stroke patients will significantly reduce the abovementioned risks. However, delirium in stroke patients is not very different from the delirium in other conditions from a clinical viewpoint, and a delay in diagnosis may be experienced particularly in patients presenting with delirium or in strokes without obvious paresis or in cases developing delirium immediately after the stroke. Another potential reason for this delay in the diagnosis of delirium is the fluctuating clinical course, and if a diagnosis of delirium is overlooked, the risk of death may be increased up to eightfold, particularly among the elderly. Therefore, clinicians caring for such patients should be encouraged to use the validated tests for delirium to detect the early signs, and the chance of administering treatment in the early course of the disease should not be missed. In a study examining the causes of delayed diagnosis in delirium, the following four independent risk factors were identified: hypoactive delirium, age equal to or greater than 80 years, presence of visual disturbance, and presence of dementia. If none of these risk factors are present, the risk of delirium is 2%, while the risk increases to 6%, 15%, and 44% with 1, 2, and 3 or 4 risk factors, respectively. In other words, the risk of overlooking a diagnosis of delirium in the presence of ≥ three risk factors is 20-fold higher (Inouye et al. 2001; Baddeley et al. 1995). Thus, patients with any of these four risk factors should be more closely observed for the signs and symptoms of delirium. Also other factors such as the possible development of neglect, aphasia, or dysphagia may complicate the assessment of delirium, and currently no consensus exists on this issue. Similarly, there are no well-defined diagnostic criteria that are widely used to diagnose poststroke delirium.

Delirium, particularly developing in the acute period, is an independent risk factor for the demential process that will develop within the next 2 years (van Rijsbergen et al. 2011). In such patients, multiple cognitive areas, mainly memory and visual-spatial skills, are involved. However, no clear explanations have been put forward until now for the development of such a cognitive defect. Unfortunately, very little data exists as to the outcome of the poststroke delirium and particularly the long-term effect. Although data for the timing, i.e., day, of the occurrence of delirium after an episode of stroke is limited, a previous study reported an average duration of 6.7 days (min, 2; max, 17) (Cummings 1995).

Similarly, despite the absence of adequate number of studies for the prevention of delirium after stroke, it is generally thought that delirium may actually be prevented in more than a third of the patients admitted (Inouye et al. 1999). Systemic protocols are required for the early recognition, prevention, and—if needed—treatment of patients at an increased risk of delirium in stroke units, since recovery is possible in the majority of the cases within 4 weeks or earlier when an early diagnosis is accomplished with appropriate treatment, particularly when the underlying disorder is corrected (Brown et al. 2011). The primary target in the assessment of delirium developing in stroke patients is to evaluate the potential metabolic causes. Although it is not significantly different from the current treatments for delirium, treatment with rivastigmine, a cholinesterase inhibitor, has been associated with good response rates (Oldenbeuving et al. 2008).

### 7.8.2 Delirium in Dementia

Dementia is a disorder characterized by a significant disturbance in cognitive abilities that leads to an adverse effect on activities of daily living. Similar types of disturbances occur at varying degrees in delirium as well. Although there are many symptoms common to both of these conditions, significant differences also exist with respect to the etiopathogenesis, diagnostic procedures, presentation and duration of the disease, clinical course, therapeutic approaches, type of the involvement of cognitive functions, and sleep-wakefulness cycle, and a failure to timely intervene may increase the risk of morbidity and mortality, particularly in patients with delirium. Delirium in dementia is detailed at the chapter entitled "Delirium Superimposed Dementia" in this book.

### 7.8.3 Delirium in Encephalopathy

Encephalopathy is a neurological syndrome characterized by motor or mental dysfunction occurring due to injury or functional impairment of the brain tissue as a result of a variety of conditions. Encephalopathy itself does not represent a single entity but rather can be considered as a collection of a wide range of symptoms from a mild personality disorder to dementia, epilepsy, delirium, coma, and even death. Many reasons, such as infectious, hepatic, uremic, ischemic, metabolic (hyper-/hypocalcemia, hyper-/hyponatremia, hyper-/hypoglycemia), malnutrition, and toxic substances may cause encephalopathy.

A proper balance between electrolytes, amino acids, excitatory and inhibitory neurotransmitters, and oxygen supply is required for normal neuronal activity (McCusker et al. 2001). Also blood flow, temperature, osmolality, and pH should be within the normal limits for optimum functions of the CNS. This balance is necessary for normal cognitive functions, wakefulness, ascending reticular activating system (ARAS), and its projections in the cerebral cortex (Earnest and Parker 1993). Encephalopathic delirium refers to a change in the mental state occurring due to the abovementioned derangements in different types of encephalopathy. Frequently, it is accompanied by fluctuations in the consciousness, hallucinations, impaired orientation, and memory problems.

Patients with encephalopathy are frequently admitted to specific units, although some patients present directly with delirium. In fact, in patients with no previously known conditions presenting with delirium, encephalopathy should always be considered in the differential diagnosis with appropriate investigations. After obtaining a detailed history from the caregivers, a general physical and neurological examination should be performed, followed by rapid assessment of laboratory parameters such as the metabolic panel, complete blood count, liver function tests, ammonia level, vitamin B1 level, calcium level, thyroid function tests, urinalysis, toxicology, and HIV test, and subsequently a cranial imaging study, preferably with contrast enhancement, should be scheduled.

Encephalopathies do not exhibit a specific presentation of delirium, and clinically the two conditions may frequently have similarities. However, certain encephalopathic conditions have a more specific clinical course, providing clues for early diagnosis and treatment. For instance, while pupillary responses are preserved in metabolic encephalopathy, it is lost in Wernicke's or hepatic encephalopathy, particularly in the advanced stages. Another type of encephalopathy, which is frequently confused with stroke and treated accordingly, is represented by the focal neurological deficit commonly seen in both hypo- and hyperglycemia encephalopathies. Wernicke's encephalopathy results from vitamin B1 deficiency and is characterized by encephalopathy, gait ataxia, ophthalmoparesis, and nystagmus. The most common and initial clinical sign is mental confusion, followed by ataxia and eye signs. Although Wernicke's encephalopathy sometimes may start with mild confusion, very severe delirium is also not uncommon. Failure to administer timely and adequate treatment results in Korsakoff amnestic syndrome and even coma and death.

Standard diagnostic delirium tools (CAM or CAM-ICU) may also be used in encephalopathic patients with delirium. Also specific pathological wave patterns of

EEG are common in patients with encephalopathy. For instance, triphasic waves are seen in metabolic encephalopathy with marked rhythmic delta activity, particularly in the frontal areas. However, in patients with a suspicion of encephalopathy, continuous EEG monitoring is very important for the assessment of nonconvulsive episodes, regardless of the development of delirium (Plum and Posner 1982). Standard diagnostic tools used in delirium may be used delirium induced by encephalopathy.

In patients admitted to an intensive care unit who have treatment-resistant encephalopathy, a possibility of delirium should be borne in mind. Particularly, in patients with prolonged delirium, there are certain risks such as increased duration of hospital stay, mechanical ventilation, and nosocomial infection, which ultimately increase the risk of morbidity and mortality (İnouye et al. 1998).

### 7.8.4 Delirium in Other Neurologic Disorders

As stated above, many neurological conditions, particularly those directly involving the CNS, are associated with an increased risk of delirium. Delirium developing on such a background does not exhibit a specific clinical pattern, and frequently, delirium is preceded by the clinical signs and symptoms of the underlying condition.

Delirium may also develop during the course of an acute or chronic infection involving the parenchyma of the CNS or meningeal tissue. There is a particularly increased risk of delirium in encephalitis involving the temporal lobes.

Transient global amnesia (TGA) is a rare neurological condition of acute onset characterized by anterograde and retrograde amnesia, confusion, and anxiety mostly occurring in the middle-aged individuals. It is generally a spontaneously occurring condition, although it may sometimes occur after a minor head trauma, excessive fatigue, or emotional stress. Emergence of confusion during the course of TGA may lead to delirium when combined with the effects of anxiety.

Psychotic symptoms may occur during the course of idiopathic Parkinson's disease (IPD) or as a side effect of the medications used for treatment. While the degeneration of the dopaminergic neurons in the substantia nigra is associated with the specific motor symptoms of IPD such as bradykinesia, rigidity, and tremors, the dopaminergic degeneration in the midbrain and the ventral tegmental area may cause psychomotor retardation, anxiety, depression, and impaired cognitive functions. IPD is not only associated with dopaminergic losses but also with cholinergic and serotonergic losses, leading to cognitive impairment and psychotic symptoms. Also, psychotic signs of İPH may exhibit a bimodal course. In other words, while they may be associated with the motor fluctuations and dopaminergic medications in the early stages, they result from the cognitive impairment in the later stages (Wolters and Berendese 2001).

Another condition that should be considered in the differential diagnosis of delirium is posterior reversible encephalopathy syndrome (PRES), which is characterized by confusion, epilepsy, loss of vision, and psychotic symptoms, which can be diagnosed by typical radiological findings and which can usually be reversed by the removal of the causative factors.

## References

Allen SJ, MacGowan SH, Tyler S et al (1997) Reduced cholinergic function in normal and Alzheimer's disease brain is associated with apolipoprotein E4 genotype. Neurosci Lett 239:33–36

American Psychiatric Association (2000) Diagnostic and statistical manual of mental disorders (text revision), 4th edn. American Psychiatric Association, Washington, DC

Baddeley A, Wilson B, Watts F (eds) (1995) Handbook of memory disorders. Wiley, Chichester

Breitbart W, Cohen K (2000) Delirium in the terminally ill. In: Chochinov H, Breitbart W (eds) Handbook of psychiatry in palliative medicine. Oxford University Press, New York, pp 75–90

Broadhurst C, Wilson K (2001) Immunology of delirium: new opportunities for treatment and research. Br J Psychiatry 179:288–289

Brodaty H, Ames D, Snowdon J et al (2003) A randomized placebo-controlled trial of risperidone for the treatment of aggression, agitation, and psychosis of dementia. J Clin Psychiatry 64:134–143

Brown LJ, Fordyce C, Zaghdani H et al (2011) Detecting deficits of sustained visual attention in delirium. J Neurol Neurosurg Psychiatry 82:1334–1340

Caeiro L, Ferro JM, Albuquerque R, Figueira ML (2004) Delirium in the first days of acute stroke. J Neurol 251:171–178

Cole MG, McCusker J, Bellavance F et al (2002) Systematic detection and multidisciplinary care of delirium in older medical inpatients: a randomized trial.[see comment]. Can Med Assoc J 167(7):753–759

Cole MG (2004) Delirium in elderly patients. Am J Geriatr Psychiatry 12:7–21

Cummings J (1995) Neuropsychiatry. In: Simpson MG (ed) Psychiatric disorders. Impact Communications, New York, pp 109–136

De Deyn PP, Rabheru K, Rasmussen A et al (1999) A randomized trial of risperidone, placebo, and haloperidol for behavioral symptoms of dementia. Neurology 53:946–955

Earnest MP, Parker WD (1993) Metabolic encephalopathies and coma from medical causes. In: Grotta J (ed) Management of the acutely ill neurological patient. Churchill Livingstone, New York, p 1

Ely EW, Shintani A, Truman B et al (2004) Delirium as a predictor of mortality in mechanically ventilated patients in the intensive care unit. JAMA 291(14):1753–1762

Engel GL, Romano J (2004) Delirium, a syndrome of cerebral insufficiency. J Neuropsychiatry Clin Neurosci 16(4):526–538

Flacker JM, Cummings V, Mach JR Jr et al (1998) The association of serum anticholinergic activity with delirium in elderly medical patients. Am J Geriatr Psychiatry 6:31–41

Fong TG, Bogardus ST Jr, Daftary A et al (2006) Cerebral perfusion changes in older delirious patients using 99mTc HMPAO SPECT. J Gerontol A Biol Sci Med Sci 61:1294–1299

Gustafson Y, Olsson T, Asplund K, Hägg E (1993) Acute confusional state (delirium) soon after stroke is associated with hypercortisolism. Cerebrovasc Dis 3:33

Gustafson Y, Olsson T, Erikkson S, Bucht G (1991) Acute confusional state (delirium) in stroke patients. Cerebrovasc Dis 1:257–264

Hales E, Yudofsky JA (eds) (2003) The American Psychiatric Press textbook of psychiatry. American Psychiatric Publishing, Washington, DC

Henon H, Lebert F, Durieu I et al (1999) Confusional state in stroke: relation to preexisting dementia, patient characteristics, and outcome. Stroke 30:773–779

Inao S, Kawai T, Kabeya R et al (2001) Relation between brain displacement and local cerebral blood flow in patients with chronic subdural haematoma. J Neurol Neurosurg Psychiatry 71:741–746

Inouye SK, Bogardus ST, Charpentier PA et al (1999) A multicomponent intervention to prevent delirium in hospitalized older patients. N Engl J Med 340:669–676

Inouye SK, Foreman MD, Mion LC et al (2001) Nurses' recognition of delirium and its symptoms: comparison of nurse and researcher ratings. Arch Intern Med 161:2467–2473

Inouye S, van Dyck C, Alessi C (1990) Clarifying confusion: the confusion assessment method. Ann Intern Med 113(12):941–948
İnouye SK, Rushing JT, Foreman MD et al (1998) Does delirium contribute to poor hospital outcomes? A three-site epidemiologic study. J Gen Intern Med 13(4):234–242
Jacobson S, Jerrier H (2000) EEG in delirium. Semin Clin Neuropsychiatry 5:86–92
Langhorne P, Stott DJ, Robertson L et al (2000) Medical complications after stroke: a multicenter study. Stroke 31(6):1223–1229
Lipowski ZJ (1990) Delirium: acute confusional states. Oxford University Press, New York
Maldonado JR (2008) Pathoetiological model of delirium: a comprehensive understanding of the neurobiology of delirium and an evidence-based approach to prevention and treatment. Crit Care Clin 24:789–856
McCusker J, Cole M, Dendukuri N et al (2001) Delirium in older medical inpatients and subsequent cognitive and functional status: a prospective study. CMAJ 165:575–583
Meagher DJ, O'Hanlon D, O'Mahony E et al (2000) Relationship between symptoms and motoric subtype of delirium. J Neuropsychiatr Clin Neurosci 12(1):51–56
Milstein A, Arak Y, Kleinman G et al (2001) The incidence of delirium immediately following cataract removal surgery: a prospective study in the elderly. Aging Mental Health 4:178–181
Oldenbeuving AW, de Kort PLM, Jansen BPW et al (2011) Delirium in the acute phase after stroke: incidence, risk factors, and outcome. Neurology 76:993–999
Oldenbeuving AW, de Kort PL, Jansen BP et al (2008) A pilot study of rivastigmine in the treatment of delirium after stroke: a safe alternative. BMC Neurol 8:34
Plum F, Posner JB (1982) The diagnosis of stupor and coma. FA Davis Company, Philadelphia, p 177
Rechtschaffen A, Kales A (1968) A manual of standardized terminology, techniques, and scoring system for sleep stages of human subjects. U.S. Government Printing Office, Washington, DC
van Rijsbergen MWA, Oldenbeuving AW, Nieuwenhuis-Mark RE et al (2011) Delirium in acute stroke: a predictor of subsequent cognitive impairment? A two-year follow-up study. J Neurol Sci 306:138–142
Schuurmans MJ, Deschamps PI, Markham SW, Shortridge-Baggett LM, Duursma SA (2003) The measurement of delirium: review of scales. Res Theory Nurs Pract 17(3):207–224
Sharon K, Inouye SK (2006) Delirium in older persons. N Engl J Med 354:1157–1165
Sheng AZ, Shen Q, Cordato D et al (2006) Delirium within three days of stroke in a cohort of elderly patients. J Am Geriatr Soc 54:1192–1198
Siddiq N, House A, Holmes J (2006) Occurrence and outcome of delirium in medical in-patients: a systematic literature review. Age Aging 35:350–364
Street JS, Clark WS, Gannon KS et al (2000) Olanzapine treatment of psychotic and behavioral symptoms in patients with Alzheimer disease in nursing care facilities: a double-blind, randomized, placebo-controlled trial. The HGEU Study Group. Arch Gen Psychiatry 57:968–976
Thomas C, Hestermann U, Kopitz J et al (2008) Serum anticholinergic activity and cerebral cholinergic dysfunction: an EEG study in frail elderly with and without delirium. BMC Neurosci 86:1–10
Trzepacz P, Mittal D, Torres R et al (2001) Validation of the delirium rating scale-revised-98: comparison with the Delirium Rating Scale and the Cognitive Test for Delirium. J Neuropsychiatry Clin Neurosci 13:229–242
Trzepacz PT (2000) Is there a final common neural pathway in delirium? Focus on acetylcholine and dopamine. Semin Clin Neuropsychiatry 5:132–148
Van Munster BC, Korevaar JC, Zwinderman AH et al (2009) The association between delirium and the apolipoprotein E epsilon 4 allele: new study results and a meta-analysis. Am J Geriatr Psychiatry 17:856–862
Wolters EC, Berendese HW (2001) Management of psychosis in Parkinson's disease. Curr Op Neurol 14:499–504
Young J, Inouye SK (2007) Delirium in older people. BMJ 334:842–846

# 8 Approach to the Elderly Patient with Delirium: The Intensive Care Specialist's Perspective

Yusuf Savran and Bilgin Comert

Delirium is accepted as an acute organ dysfunction in intensive care units (ICU). There is an acute deterioration in consciousness and cognition with fluctuations, and main characteristics of delirium are defined by the American Psychiatry Association in the DSM-5 (American Psychiatric Association 2013).

Delirium in the elderly is a frequent condition in ICU. It can be seen in 60–80% of the patients on mechanical ventilation support, while this proportion is lower (20–50%) in the patients not on mechanical ventilation (Ely et al. 2001a, b; Dubois et al. 2001; Girard et al. 2008; Pandharipande et al. 2007, 2008). Delirium has marked negative effects on short- and long-term results of the patients. The patients with delirium in ICU are at increased risk of undesirable conditions like prolonged mechanical ventilation, catheter removal, self-extubation, and need for physical restraints (Girard et al. 2008; Micek et al. 2005; Shehabi et al. 2010). Additionally, delirium causes longer hospital stays, more treatment costs, increased inhospital mortality risk, and increased necessity of nursing home care after discharge (Shehabi et al. 2010; Ely et al. 2001a, b, 2004; Ouimet et al. 2007; Thomason et al. 2005; Milbrandt et al. 2004; Inouye and Charpentier 1996).

The common misconception is that delirious patients have either hallucination or delusion. These symptoms are not necessary for diagnosis. Other frequent symptoms seen in patients with delirium are sleep disturbances, abnormal psychomotor activity, and emotional disturbances (e.g., fear, anxiety, depression, apathy, euphoria, anger). Patients with delirium may be agitated (hyperactive delirium) and calm or lethargic (hypoactive delirium) or may fluctuate in between these two types. While hallucination and delusions frequently accompany hyperactive delirium, hypoactive delirium generally is characterized with confusion and sedation (Barr et al. 2013).

Y. Savran, M.D. • B. Comert, M.D. (✉)
Department of Medical Intensive Care Unit, School of Medicine, Dokuz Eylül University, Izmir, Turkey
e-mail: bilgincomert@yahoo.com



A.T. Isik, G.T. Grossberg (eds.), *Delirium in Elderly Patients*,
https://doi.org/10.1007/978-3-319-65239-9_8

Since delirium is frequent in ICU and has negative effects on outcome, avoiding occurrence of delirium is a key factor for increasing ICU care quality. Only one factor may be responsible of delirium while sometimes it may be multifactorial. Mostly the factor causing delirium is the indication for ICU admission. Delirium may already be present during the period of ICU admission. Correcting the problem causing delirium and eliminating other risk factors for delirium will provide the condition to ameliorate in a shorter span of time.

## 8.1 Risk Factors for Delirium in ICU

In a mean medical ICU patient, there are 11 or more risk factors for delirium (Ely et al. 2001a, b). Risk factors may be classified as preexisting condition, acute illness-related, and hospital-related (treatment and ICU environment) factors (Table 8.1) (Inouye and Charpentier 1996; Brummel and Girard 2013). These factors assembling together cause delirium to become overt as in elderly patients. In a sensitive person, such as an elderly patient with dementia, a simple urinary tract

**Table 8.1** Risk factors for delirium

| |
|---|
| *Preexisting conditions* |
| • Age > 70 years |
| • Loss of sensation (visual or hearing) |
| • Transfer from a nursing home |
| • History of depression, dementia, cardiac insufficiency, stroke, epilepsy |
| • Renal or liver disease |
| • Alcohol or drug abuse |
| • Use of psychotropic drugs (anticholinergics, benzodiazepines, opiates) |
| • Malnutrition |
| *Acute illness related* |
| • High severity of illness |
| • Metabolic disturbances (glycemia, natremia, azotemia, etc.) |
| • Hypothermia or fever |
| • Sepsis, ARDS |
| • Need for mechanical ventilation |
| • Anemia |
| • Acidosis |
| • Hypotension |
| *Hospital (ICU) related* |
| • Medications (anticholinergics, sedatives, analgesics) |
| • Number of used medications |
| • Immobility, physical restrains |
| • Urinary and vascular catheters |
| • Gastric tubes |
| • Sleep deprivation |
| • Lack of daylight |
| • Isolation, lack of visitors |

infection may predispose delirium, while in a less sensitive person, such as a young patient without predisposing factors, septic shock, and acute respiratory distress syndrome (ARDS), mechanical ventilation support may cause delirium.

## 8.2 Detection of Delirium

Delirium is a frequent problem in ICU patients whether on mechanical ventilation or not (Ely et al. 2013; Dubois et al. 2001; Girard et al. 2008; Micek et al. 2005; Bergeron et al. 2001). Since hypoactive delirium is more frequent than hyperactive one, it is generally underdiagnosed by ICU staff (Peterson et al. 2006). Delirium can be detected in intubated and spontaneous breathing patients by tools proven to be valid and safe. Trials with these tools showed that patients with delirium could be detected successfully, and using these tools routinely in ICU increased quality (Spronk et al. 2009). Patients with medium- and high-risk factors for delirium (alcoholism, cognitive dysfunction, hypertension, severe sepsis or septic shock, mechanical ventilation, parenteral sedative and opiate infusion) should be screened at least once in every nursing shift with a valid and safe delirium assessment tool.

In a meta-analysis of delirium screening tools in ICU, Confusion Assessment Method for the Intensive Care Unit [CAM-ICU] and Intensive Care Delirium Screening Checklist [ICDSC] were found to be the most sensitive and specific screening tools (Neto et al. 2012).

It was shown that screening for delirium is practical in clinics. In multicenter trials, more than 2000 patients showed delirium monitoring compliance rates in excess of 90% (Barr et al. 2013).

## 8.3 Prevention of Delirium

The preventive measures for delirium should be patient specific because risk factors have individual variations. Nevertheless, due to the routine applications in ICU, sedative usage, immobility, and sleep disorders are common problems and potential targets in preventing delirium (Brummel and Girard 2013).

### 8.3.1 Sedative Usage

Using sedatives in mechanically ventilated patients in ICU is a worldwide application (Patel et al. 2009). To prevent delirium and improve brain functions, two basic points about using sedatives stand out: first, daily withholding sedatives to awaken the patients and applying spontaneous breathing trials and, second, trying to avoid using benzodiazepines.

In Awakening and Breathing Controlled (ABC) trial, daily withholding sedatives, and applying spontaneous breathing trials in either continuous infusion or intermittent bolus group, it was shown that days of acute brain dysfunction of the patients were significantly less when compared to the control group (Girard et al. 2008).

In most of the trials conducted in various ICU clinics, benzodiazepines were found to be associated with delirium. Pandharipande et al. reported lorazepam usage is related with the risk of developing delirium the next day in a dose-dependent manner (Pandharipande et al. 2006). Almost all of the patients receiving 20 mg and more lorazepam (except comatose patients that could not be assessed for delirium) were found to have delirium the next day. A trial conducted in a surgical and trauma ICU reported 2.75-fold increased risk of delirium in patients treated with midazolam (Pandharipande et al. 2008). Therefore, one of the precautions to prevent delirium in ICU is avoiding the use of benzodiazepines for routine sedation.

Dexmedetomidine usage in ICU may reduce the risk of delirium. Pandharipande et al. compared the effect of dexmedetomidine on delirium with that of lorazepam (MENDS, Maximizing the Efficacy of Targeted Sedation and Reducing Neurologic Dysfunction) in a randomized, double-blind, multicenter study. They found that patients receiving dexmedetomidine had significantly more coma-free and delirium-free days than patients using lorazepam (Pandharipande et al. 2007). In another randomized, double-blind, multicenter study (DEXCOM), the incidence of delirium did not significantly differ, although the duration of delirium was significantly shorter in patients using dexmedetomidine compared with patients using morphine (Shehabi et al. 2009). In a randomized, open-label, single center study, the incidence of delirium in patients treated with dexmedetomidine was significantly less than patients treated with remifentanil (Park et al. 2014). In another randomized, open-label, single center study, the incidence of delirium in patients treated with dexmedetomidine was significantly less than patients treated with propofol or midazolam (Maldonado et al. 2009).

### 8.3.2 Management of Pain

Pain is an evitable risk factor for delirium and inadequate management of pain in ICU is a common cause for agitation. An incorrect application in ICU is neglecting pain screening and treatment and using sedatives inadequately instead of analgesics. Payen et al. reported less consumption of sedatives, especially benzodiazepines which increase the risk for delirium and more consumption of analgesics (opiates and non-opiates) when ICU patients were regularly screened for pain (Payen et al. 2009). The dual effect of opiates having both analgesic and sedative properties should not be neglected. Opiates, when used for analgesia in ICU patients, decrease the risk of delirium (Pandharipande et al. 2008).But there is significant data that opiates may trigger delirium when used in high doses for sedation (Ouimet et al. 2007; Pisani et al. 2009). Therefore, regular pain screening and avoiding deep sedation with high doses of opiates in ICU patients are recommended.

### 8.3.3 Early Mobilization

Many trials outside ICU reported immobility to be a risk factor for delirium (Inouye and Charpentier 1996). In the past, it was believed that ICU patients, especially those receiving mechanical ventilation, are not appropriate for physical rehabilitation and mobilization. But recently, this belief has significantly changed, and many reports showed that physical rehabilitation and mobilization are effective and safe during the early phases of treatment in ICU patients (Bailey et al. 2007; Schweickert et al. 2009; Needham et al. 2010).

In a randomized controlled trial by Schweickert et al., physical rehabilitation and mobilization were applied to patients in the first 72 h after endotracheal intubation, and they were screened daily for delirium (Schweickert et al. 2009). In the patients who underwent physical rehabilitation and mobilization in the early phase, delirium period was 50% less than the standard treatment group. Similar results were reached in a quality improvement project of Johns Hopkins Hospital during decrementing deep sedation and increasing patients' mobility in the early phase (Needham et al. 2010). In the year after the quality improvement project was put into practice, when compared to previous years, the patient days spent in delirium and comatose state decreased. These findings indicate that early mobilization of ICU patients is effective in reducing delirium periods.

### 8.3.4 Improving Sleep

Sleep disturbances are common among ICU patients; they sleep 2–8 h of 24 h in average (Needham et al. 2010). Half of the time spent in sleep in ICU is during the daytime hours and interrupted frequently, REM period is short, and the sleep is not restful and restorative (Cooper et al. 2000; Gabor et al. 2003). There are many factors interrupting sleep in ICU environment. These are the alarms of devices, light, noise of the staff, treatment applications, pain, anxiety, and ventilator dyssynchrony. Additionally, the patients' treatment frequently includes sedatives (especially benzodiazepines), analgesics, vasopressors, β-agonists, and corticosteroids which interrupt the REM period of sleep (Bourne and Mills 2004). The relation between insomnia and delirium is not clear because both of them share the same symptoms. Van Rompaey et al. randomized patients into two groups and used earplug in the study group during nighttime. The patients with earplug stated that they slept better on the first night in ICU, and during 5 days of the trial, less patients in this group experienced delirium or minimal confusion (Van Rompaey et al. 2012).

Strategies to diminish noise in ICU (earplug), organize day and night lightening, and minimize treatment applications during sleep and attempts to improve patient comfort are generally inexpensive and nonhazardous efforts to be used for prevention of delirium.

### 8.3.5 Pharmacologic Interventions

Presently, there is no pharmacologic agent approved by FDA for prevention of delirium. There are few randomized controlled trials about the role of antipsychotic agents in the prevention of delirium. In a multicenter trial, MIND (Modifying the Incidence of Neurologic Dysfunction) patients on mechanical ventilation were randomized into three groups and treated with haloperidol, ziprasidone, or placebo, respectively. When compared to placebo, none of the antipsychotic agents improved the period of normal brain function (Girard et al. 2010). On the other hand, Wang et al. randomized patients over 65 years of age undergone noncardiac surgery postoperatively into haloperidol and placebo groups and at the end of 7-day trial reported less delirium in haloperidol group (Wang et al. 2012). The most important difference between these two trials was the severity of diseases of the patients included. While the patients in the trial of Wang et al. were elective surgery patients, in MIND study, mechanically ventilated patients with acute respiratory distress syndrome were included. Since now, only these two studies are placebo controlled trials investigating the effect of antipsychotic agents in the prevention of delirium. In a before/after observation study by Boogaard et al. after prophylaxis with haloperidol, there was a decrease in the incidence of delirium and an increase in delirium-free days (van den Boogaard et al. 2013). There is a need for more evidence to recommend the routine use of antipsychotic agents for prevention of delirium in ICU.

## 8.4 Treatment of Delirium

Although there is no proof of a double-blinded, randomized, and placebo controlled trial stating the efficiency and safety of any antipsychotic agent in the treatment of delirium, many international guidelines recommend the use of antipsychotic agents, and these agents are used by many intensivists in the treatment of delirium in ICU (Martin et al. 2010; Potter and George 2006). The proof level of using haloperidol for delirium in ICU patients is only level C (observational trials). There is no newly published prospective trial indicating the efficacy and safety of haloperidol for the treatment of delirium in ICU.

There are limited number of studies evaluating the treatment of delirium. In the MIND (Modifying the Incidence of Delirium) trial, there was no difference in delirium-free days in patients with haloperidol, ziprasidone, or placebo (Girard et al. 2010). There is also no recommendation of antipsychotic agents to be used in ICU patients by Cochrane Review (Lonergan et al. 2007).

## References

American Psychiatric Association (2013) DSM-5 Task Force. Diagnostic and statistical manual of mental disorders: DSM-5. American Psychiatric Association, Washington, DC

Bailey P, Thomsen GE, Spuhler VJ et al (2007) Early activity is feasible and safe in respiratory failure patients. Crit Care Med 35(1):139–145

Barr J, Fraser GL, Puntillo K et al (2013) Clinical practice guidelines for the management of pain, agitation, and delirium in adult patients in the intensive care unit. Crit Care Med 41(1):263–306

Bergeron N, Dubois MJ, Dumont M et al (2001) Intensive care delirium screening checklist: evaluation of a new screening tool. Intensive Care Med 27(5):859–864

Bourne RS, Mills GH (2004) Sleep disruption in critically ill patients-pharmacological considerations. Anaesthesia 59(4):374–384

Brummel NE, Girard TD (2013) Preventing delirium in the intensive care unit. Crit Care Clin 29(1):51–65

Cooper AB, Thornley KS, Young GB et al (2000) Sleep in critically ill patients requiring mechanical ventilation. Chest 117(3):809–818

Dubois MJ, Bergeron N, Dumont M et al (2001) Delirium in an intensive care unit: a study of risk factors. Intensive Care Med 27(8):1297–1304

Ely EW, Gautam S, Margolin R et al (2001a) The impact of delirium in the intensive care unit on hospital length of stay. Intensive Care Med 27(12):1892–1900

Ely EW, Inouye SK, Bernard GR et al (2001b) Delirium in mechanically ventilated patients: validity and reliability of the confusion assessment method for the intensive care unit (CAM-ICU). JAMA 286(21):2703–2710

Ely EW, Shintani A, Truman B et al (2004) Delirium as a predictor of mortality in mechanically ventilated patients in the intensive care unit. JAMA 291(14):1753–1762

Gabor JY, Cooper AB, Crombach SA et al (2003) Contribution of the intensive care unit environment to sleep disruption in mechanically ventilated patients and healthy subjects. Am J Respir Crit Care Med 167(5):708–715

Girard TD, Kress JP, Fuchs BD et al (2008) Efficacy and safety of a paired sedation and ventilator weaning protocol for mechanically ventilated patients in intensive care (Awakening and Breathing Controlled trial): a randomised controlled trial. Lancet 371(9607):126–134

Girard TD, Pandharipande PP, Carson SS et al (2010) Feasibility, efficacy, and safety of antipsychotics for intensive care unit delirium: the MIND randomized, placebo-controlled trial. Crit Care Med 38(2):428–437

Hsieh SJ, Ely EW, Gong MN (2013) Can intensive care unit delirium be prevented and reduced? Lessons learned and future directions. Ann Am Thorac Soc 10(6):648–56

Inouye SK, Charpentier PA (1996) Precipitating factors for delirium in hospitalized elderly persons. Predictive model and interrelationship with baseline vulnerability. JAMA 275(11): 852–857

Lonergan E, Britton AM, Luxenberg J et al (2007) Antipsychotics for delirium. Cochrane Database Syst Rev (2):CD005594

Maldonado JR, Wysong A, van der Starre PJ et al (2009) Dexmedetomidine and the reduction of postoperative delirium after cardiac surgery. Psychosomatics 50(3):206–217

Martin J, Heymann A, Basell K et al (2010) Evidence and consensus-based German guidelines for the management of analgesia, sedation and delirium in intensive care—short version. Ger Med Sci 8:Doc02

Micek ST, Anand NJ, Laible BR et al (2005) Delirium as detected by the CAM-ICU predicts restraint use among mechanically ventilated medical patients. Crit Care Med 33(6): 1260–1265

Milbrandt EB, Deppen S, Harrison PL et al (2004) Costs associated with delirium in mechanically ventilated patients. Crit Care Med 32(4):955–962

Needham DM, Korupolu R, Zanni JM et al (2010) Early physical medicine and rehabilitation for patients with acute respiratory failure: a quality improvement project. Arch Phys Med Rehabil 91(4):536–542

Neto AS, Nassar AP Jr, Cardoso SO et al (2012) Delirium screening in critically ill patients: a systematic review and meta-analysis. Crit Care Med 40(6):1946–1951

Ouimet S, Kavanagh BP, Gottfried SB et al (2007) Incidence, risk factors and consequences of ICU delirium. Intensive Care Med 33(1):66–73

Pandharipande P, Shintani A, Peterson J et al (2006) Lorazepam is an independent risk factor for transitioning to delirium in intensive care unit patients. Anesthesiology 104(1):21–26

Pandharipande PP, Pun BT, Herr DL et al (2007) Effect of sedation with dexmedetomidine vs lorazepam on acute brain dysfunction in mechanically ventilated patients: the MENDS randomized controlled trial. JAMA 298(22):2644–2653

Pandharipande P, Cotton BA, Shintani A et al (2008) Prevalence and risk factors for development of delirium in surgical and trauma intensive care unit patients. J Trauma 65(1):34–41

Park JB, Bang SH, Chee HK et al (2014) Efficacy and safety of dexmedetomidine for postoperative delirium in adult cardiac surgery on cardiopulmonary bypass. Korean J Thorac Cardiovasc Surg 47(3):249–254
Patel RP, Gambrell M, Speroff T et al (2009) Delirium and sedation in the intensive care unit: survey of behaviors and attitudes of 1384 healthcare professionals. Crit Care Med 37(3): 825–832
Payen JF, Bosson JL, Chanques G et al (2009) Pain assessment is associated with decreased duration of mechanical ventilation in the intensive care unit: a post Hoc analysis of the DOLOREA study. Anesthesiology 111(6):1308–1316
Peterson JF, Pun BT, Dittus RS et al (2006) Delirium and its motoric subtypes: a study of 614 critically ill patients. J Am Geriatr Soc 54(3):479–484
Pisani MA, Murphy TE, Araujo KL et al (2009) Benzodiazepine and opioid use and the duration of intensive care unit delirium in an older population. Crit Care Med 37(1):177–183
Potter J, George J (2006) The prevention, diagnosis and management of delirium in older people: concise guidelines. Clin Med 6(3):303–308
Schweickert WD, Pohlman MC, Pohlman AS et al (2009) Early physical and occupational therapy in mechanically ventilated, critically ill patients: a randomised controlled trial. Lancet 373(9678):1874–1882
Shehabi Y, Grant P, Wolfenden H et al (2009) Prevalence of delirium with dexmedetomidine compared with morphine based therapy after cardiac surgery: a randomized controlled trial (DEXmedetomidine COmpared to Morphine-DEXCOM Study). Anesthesiology 111(5):1075–1084
Shehabi Y, Riker RR, Bokesch PM et al (2010) Delirium duration and mortality in lightly sedated, mechanically ventilated intensive care patients. Crit Care Med 38(12):2311–2318
Spronk PE, Riekerk B, Hofhuis J et al (2009) Occurrence of delirium is severely underestimated in the ICU during daily care. Intensive Care Med 35(7):1276–1280
Thomason JW, Shintani A, Peterson JF et al (2005) Intensive care unit delirium is an independent predictor of longer hospital stay: a prospective analysis of 261 non-ventilated patients. Crit Care 9(4):R375–R381
van den Boogaard M, Schoonhoven L, van Achterberg T et al (2013) Haloperidol prophylaxis in critically ill patients with a high risk for delirium. Crit Care 17(1):R9
Van Rompaey B, Elseviers MM, Van Drom W et al (2012) The effect of earplugs during the night on the onset of delirium and sleep perception: a randomized controlled trial in intensive care patients. Crit Care 16(3):R73
Wang W, Li HL, Wang DX et al (2012) Haloperidol prophylaxis decreases delirium incidence in elderly patients after noncardiac surgery: a randomized controlled trial*. Crit Care Med 40(3):731–739

# 9 Approach to the Elderly Patient with Delirium: Nursing Perspective

Özlem Küçükgüçlü

Delirium is a neglected condition relative to its frequency and serious consequences. Delirium is a serious, common, and potentially preventable source of morbidity and mortality in older patients. Delirium is defined as an acute fluctuating change in mental state, with consciousness and cognitive impairment. It is highly prevalent, costly, and a global problem in older adults (Steis and Fick 2007). It has a high incidence, as well as being associated with increased morbidity and mortality and prolonged stays in the intensive care unit (ICU) and in hospital. Delirium has been found to be an independent predictor of increased mortality and morbidity and increased hospital stay (Luetz et al. 2010; Ouimet et al. 2007). It is a common complication of hospitalization. Studies estimate the prevalence of delirium in hospitalized patients to be 14% to 56% and up to 70% in critically ill elderly patients (Leslie et al. 2008; McNicoll et al. 2003). Delirious patients are more likely to be discharged to a nursing home and have increased hospital mortality and longer lengths of stay (Salluh et al. 2010). Long-term effects of delirium include cognitive impairment and increased likelihood of developing or worsening dementia. Fong stated that approximately one in eight hospitalized patients with AD who develop delirium will have at least one adverse outcome, including death, institutionalization, or cognitive decline, associated with delirium (Fong et al. 2012).

Elders in whom delirium goes unrecognized have a higher 6-month mortality (Kakuma et al. 2003). In the elderly patients admitted to long-term care facilities, it was found that delirium can affect functional outcomes and that the longer the episode of delirium, the worse the functional outcome (Marcantonio et al. 2003). Clinicians often think of delirium as a transient disorder that has no permanent effect on cognition, but there is evidence to suggest that elders who become delirious will have a permanent cognitive decline because of their delirious episode. It is

Ö. Küçükgüçlü, Ph.D.
Department of Internal Medicine Nursing, Dokuz Eylul University Faculty of Nursing, İnciraltı, İzmir, Turkey
e-mail: ozlem.kguclu@deu.edu.tr


A.T. Isik, G.T. Grossberg (eds.), *Delirium in Elderly Patients*,
https://doi.org/10.1007/978-3-319-65239-9_9

often thought that delirium is reversible when its underlying causes are treated but It has been shown that a significant number of delirious older adults never return to their baseline cognitive state, particularly in the presence of preexisting dementia (Rigney 2006).

Although most articles have focused on the hospitalized elder, it is important to recognize that delirium occurs outside the acute care setting as well. Several authors have discovered an alarmingly high percentage of patients discharged from the hospital in a delirious state. In older patients admitted to a home case service, 46% were delirious, and an astonishing 50% of those patients were discharged from an acute care facility to a home in which they lived alone. There are disappointingly few studies of delirium beyond hospitalization, including delirium in the long-term care setting or home setting (Rigney 2006). Despite its clinical importance, association with increased morbidity, mortality, and health services utilization remains underrecognized, misdiagnosed as dementia or other psychiatric illnesses, and undertreated (Michaud et al. 2007).

Delirium is not easy to detect, since its diagnosis is mainly clinical. To improve patient's prognosis, importance of early diagnosis and possible prevention in the different clinical scenarios is clear. A better understanding of risk factors and causes of delirium should enable nurses to focus on patients at risk. Delirium may then be avoided through meticulous assessment and early recognition of delirium symptoms. Although many cases of delirium may be unavoidable, clinical trials provide compelling evidence that at least 30–40% of cases may be preventable. Many aspects of hospital care contribute to the development of delirium, including adverse effects of medications, complications of invasive procedures, immobilization, malnutrition, dehydration, the use of bladder catheters, and sleep deprivation (Michaud et al. 2007).

Delirium is currently included as a marker of the quality of care and patient safety by the National Quality Measures Clearinghouse of the Agency for Healthcare Research and Quality (as explained at http://www.qualitymeasures.ahrq.gov/). Higher delirium rates would be expected to correlate with lower quality of hospital care. Delirium has ranked among the top three conditions for which the quality of care needs to be improved (Sloss et al. 2000).

Veteran Affairs Delirium Working Group discussed on strategies for facilitating recognition of delirium. They stated that mental status should be considered as sixth vital sign. The working group identified seven justifications for promoting mental status as "the sixth vital sign" (Flaherty et al. 2007):

1. The brain is as sensitive and vital organ as the immune (temperature), cardiac (pulse, blood pressure), and respiratory systems (respiratory rate) for heralding that something is amiss.
2. Delirium is a common, morbid, and costly condition.
3. Healthcare professionals frequently fail to evaluate mental status, and unrecognized delirium is one example of this.
4. Communication about mental status across sites of care would improve.

5. Widespread adoption would compel clinicians to become more diligent in their evaluation of the mental status as it relates to delirium and may lead to wider use of valid and reliable instruments used to evaluate patients for delirium.
6. The morbidity associated with delirium and its underlying causes is best mitigated by early intervention.
7. The elevation of mental status assessment and care to a quality measure will be facilitated.

## 9.1 Nursing Care

Delirium (as one of the "geriatric giants"), or more precisely the prevention, early recognition, and accurate treatment of delirium, is and will continue to be of major importance in the rapidly enlarging global population of hospitalized older people. Delirium is of particular interest to the nurse. Nurses have multiple contacts with patients and therefore are in a unique position to observe changes in mental status at an early stage. Although related, the concepts of nurse knowledge of delirium, nurse recognition of delirium, and nurses' assessment and documentation of delirium in older adults are different (Steis and Fick 2007). Because of its fluctuating nature and variety of presentations, however, recognition of delirium can be difficult. Nurses must be able to recognize delirium so that the underlying etiology can be discovered and treatment can begin. Unfortunately, many cases of delirium go undiagnosed (Chan and Brennan 1999). Studies suggest nurses are missing key symptoms of delirium and performing only superficial mental status assessments. Reporting rates of nurse recognition ranging from 26 to 83% compared nurses' assessments with a standardized mental status examination and found that 72% of patients with a cognitive deficit went undetected (Steis and Fick 2007). Eden and Foreman (1996) reported that lack of knowledge about assessment methods in detecting delirium and lack of communication among nursing staff were two factors in the underrecognition of delirium. Other risk factors for underrecognition by nurses include hypoactive delirium, that is, a delirium characterized by lethargy, apathy, and withdrawal; vision impairment; and preexisting dementia. Underrecognition of delirium in the elderly is by no means unique to nursing.

If nurses have not been explicitly taught the nuances of how delirium is manifested in older adults, they cannot be expected to readily recognize it at the bedside. For nurses to recognize delirium, they need time with patients, knowledge of the key features of delirium, use of an objective instrument to guide assessment and documentation, and the support of leadership within the organization (Steis and Fick 2007).

Multicomponent interventions to prevent delirium are the most effective and should be implemented through synergistic cooperation between the various healthcare disciplines. Nurses should play a pivotal role in this, as shown by most of the intervention studies (both prevention and early recognition and treatment) (Milisen et al. 2005).

### 9.1.1 Assessment of Risk Factors

Nurses play a key role in identification of delirium using valid and reliable tools and identifying modifiable risks to improve the delirious patient's outcome. If nurses lack of a sufficient understanding of delirium symptoms delirium remans underdiagnosed (Schreier 2010). Nurses are in a unique position to improve patients' quality of care and outcomes by early recognition of delirium, determining the likely causes and providing knowledgeable care. It is recommended that due to the fluctuating nature of delirium, nurses incorporate screening into patient care at least once every 8–12 h (Van den Boogaard et al. 2009).

### 9.1.2 Assessment Measures

The availability of a valid assessment instrument is a key component of any strategy to detect delirium. Numerous assessment tools have been adapted for use, and several studies have evaluated the validity and reliability of such tools. A lack of understanding and use of assessment instrumentation reduce definitive care of the delirious older adult. Therefore, the use of assessment tools is vital to effective care of older adults.

#### 9.1.2.1 Confusion Assessment Method (CAM)

It was developed based on the *Diagnostic and Statistical Manual of Mental Disorders* DSM-IV diagnostic criteria (http://www.terapiacognitiva.eu/dwl/dsm5/DSM-IV.pdf). The following elements of mental status are captured by the CAM: level of consciousness, orientation, attention or concentration, recall impairment, language, onset of symptoms, variability of symptoms, perceptual disturbances, sleep-wake disturbance, and changes in psychomotor behavior. The patient is diagnosed with delirium when the nurse identifies that the patient has an acute onset and exhibits inattention as well as either disoriented thinking or disorientation. The CAM has been used in a variety of settings, including long-term care (Inouye et al. 1999).

#### 9.1.2.2 Confusion Assessment Tool for Intensive Care Unit (CAM-ICU)

The CAM-ICU was developed based on psychiatric expert and delirium definitions of the *Diagnostic and Statistical Manual of Mental Disorders, Third Edition* (http://www.terapiacognitiva.eu/dwl/dsm5/DSM-III.pdf), to assess delirium by nonpsychiatrists. The CAM has proven to be easy to use, reliable, and valid; it was first used in the early 1990s. The CAM addresses the following four features: (a) an acute onset of mental status change or fluctuating course, (b) inattention, (c) disorganized thinking, and (d) altered level of consciousness. The CAM had limited utility in the ICU because of the inability for use in patients who were nonverbal and/or who received mechanical ventilation. The CAM-ICU modified the validated CAM for use in those patients by using nonverbal, objective instruments. To be diagnosed as delirious (CAM-ICU positive), the participant must display features 1 and 2 and either 3 or 4. The advantages of CAM-ICU include a short time for scoring (2–5 min per patient) and its high reliability. The most important contribution of the CAM-ICU is that it does not depend on the patient being able to talk verbally to assess the delirium. Thus, the CAM-ICU has the advantages in use for those patients who cannot express himself or herself with endotracheal tubes. But the CAM-ICU needs a short visual or auditory test, and this made it difficult to use. By contrast, those instruments that depend on symptom and sign score could be popular. In addition, CAM-ICU was a point-in-time assessment, and therefore, because of the fluctuating nature of delirium, it is hard to monitor the continuous situation of patients (Ely et al. 2001).

#### 9.1.2.3 The Neelon-Champagne Confusion Assessment Scale (NEECHAM)

It is designed specifically for nurses to assess the risk of confusion through bedside observation. The instrument includes all of the elements of the CAM (cognitive and behavioral components) as well as physiologic measures (appearance, vital sign stability, oxygen saturation, and urinary continence). These variables of physical function distinguish it from the other instruments that measure delirium. This instrument contains nine items organized in three domains, with a total possible score ranging from 0 to 30. A total score of 19 or less indicates moderate to severe confusion, 20–24 indicates mild or early developing confusion, 25–26 indicates not confused but with a high risk of confusion, and 27–30 indicates not confused or normal function (Neelon et al. 1996). NEECHAM is an instrument for assessing acute confusion in hospitalized patients, particularly in the early stages. The scale can be scored with data derived during routine clinical assessments of acutely ill patients. The scale detects changes in severity of acute confusion, and testing can be repeated at frequent intervals. Data needed to score the NEECHAM can be collected during 10 min of routine patient observation and vital sign assessment. For example, in scoring item 1 (attention/alertness), nurses are asked to observe the patient's immediate responsiveness to events or cues (whether the patient responds appropriately by focusing head/eyes when the nurse enters the room or approaches the bedside or by some recognition of the nurse's role, etc.). Patients with impaired arousal may not respond to the verbal commands of item 2 (complex command processing) but may respond to visually or physically cued commands, such as showing a cup of fluid or touching a cup to the lips while asking the patient to drink. Accurate scoring of the NEECHAM requires an awareness of physical disabilities (visual, hearing, motor, etc.) that affect the patient's mode of responding to signals. Eye movements, facial expressions, or responses to touch could offer acceptable alternative data for scoring (Neelon et al. 1996).

The NEECHAM scale was developed as a nursing screening and not as a diagnostic tool. This instrument uses the daily observation skills of nurses and their standard 24-h monitoring of patient in the ICU. It could enable nurses to recognize a possible delirium in an early stage so that the treatment is possible and the behavior could be prevented. This scale showed acceptable sensitivity, specificity, and predictive values. But the NEECHAM is not easy to use; it comprises three levels including nine items, and it might lead to misunderstanding for bedside nurses because of its complexity. It can only assess those who could verbally express themselves and cannot evaluate the intubated or sedated patients (Csokasy 1999).

#### 9.1.2.4 Intensive Care Delirium Screening Checklist (ICDSC)

Intensive Care Delirium Screening Checklist can easily be applied by a clinician or a nurse in a busy critical care setting to screen all patients even when communication is compromised. The tool can be utilized quickly and helps to identify delirious patients. The ICDSC assessment evaluates the level of consciousness, inattention, disorientation, hallucinations, psychomotor activity, speech or mood disturbance, sleep disturbance, and fluctuation of symptoms (Bergeron et al. 2001).

#### 9.1.2.5 Nursing Delirium Screening Scale (Nu-DESC)

The Nu-DESC is an observational five-item scale that can be completed quickly. The Nu-DESC is a delirium screening instrument that can be easily integrated into routine care and clinical practice. It is easy to use, time-efficient, and accurate and could lead to prompt delirium recognition and treatment. The Nu-DESC shows promise as a useful concomitant delirium research tool, allowing continuous screening, symptom monitoring, and severity rating. The Nu-DESC developed by Gaudreau et al. (2005) is a delirium screening instrument that can be easily integrated into routine care and clinical practice. This scoring system is largely based on the Confusion Rating Scale. However, the Nu-DESC is a five-item scale comprising, in addition to the four items of the Confusion Rating Scale, a fifth item. The addition of psychomotor retardation as the fifth major component, as well as several other subcomponents of the Nu-DESC scoring system, gave it some resemblance of the DSM-IV. The fifth item, rating unusual psychomotor retardation, took into account medical condition (delayed responsiveness and few or no spontaneous actions/words, e.g., when the patient is prodded, reaction is deferred, and/or the patient is unarousable). This brings the maximal screening score to 10. The Nu-DESC has the sensitivity of .86 and a specificity of .87 for detecting delirium. The Nu-DESC comprises only five items, so it is easy to use, time-efficient, and accurate and could lead to prompt delirium recognition and treatment. The Nu-DESC shows promise as a useful concomitant delirium assessment tool, allowing continuous screening and symptom monitoring. It is an observational screening tool for delirium, which requires no direct patient participation and can be administered by registered nurses in only 1–2 min (Gaudreau et al. 2005).

#### 9.1.2.6 Delirium Detection Score (DDS)

The DDS is an instrument adaptable to detect severe delirium. It takes into account several criteria to assess the severity of delirium. Furthermore, it might help to start a symptom-guided therapy plan easily and immediately. Thus, the DDS could help to guide the management of the delirious ICU patients and is predictive for medication use. However, the result of one study showed DDS with low sensitivity. The reason might be that the DDS looks for agitation but not psychomotor retardation, whereas the hypoactive form of delirium is much more.

The DDS is modified from the CIWA-Ar to ICU needs and is composed of eight criteria: agitation, anxiety, hallucination, orientation, seizures, tremor, paroxysmal sweating, and altered sleep-wake rhythm. For each criterion, 0, 1, 4, or 7 points can be allocated depending on the symptoms (e.g., orientation: 0 = orientated to time, place, and personal identity and able to concentrate; 1 = not sure about time and/or place, not able to concentrate; 4 = not orientated to time and/or place; 7 = not orientated to time, place, and personal identity). A total of 56 points is possible. Compared with the CIWA-Ar, in the DDS, hallucinations account for only a maximum of 7 points. Following intubation sensations (see items tactile, auditory, and visual disturbance of the CIWA-Ar), accounting for a maximum of 21 points of 67 of the CIWA-Ar would have to be set to "0" because in this incidence it is often hardly possible to diagnose hallucinations. The sensitivity and specificity of DDS were 69 and 75%.

Analysis of consecutive measurements showed that the DDS can detect symptoms of delirium, and that can help track and assess treatment. However, delirium was detected by the DDS at the same time as the clinical diagnosis of delirium was established. The DDS is composed of several criteria (agitation, anxiety, orientation, and so on) (Otter et al. 2005).

### 9.1.3 Prevention of Delirium

Despite years of evidence revealing the risks connected with delirium development, there is still a gap between current practice and ideal processes of care, since health professionals show little sensitivity toward this morbidity. It is estimated that one-third of hospital-acquired delirium cases could be prevented with appropriate interventions. Early recognition of risk factors, signs, and symptoms understanding the predisposing and precipitating risk factors is considered the most effective way to reduce delirium incidence. Since early delirium diagnosis is the first step toward prevention and treatment, the introduction into clinical practice of validated tools for neurological monitoring is a key point of hospitalized patient care. However, daily delirium monitoring is only a part of the multidimensional approach required to prevent—and treat—delirium. Evaluation of risk factors, organizational and orientation interventions, correction of underlying metabolic/organic causes before administering any neuroactive drug, early mobilization and rehabilitation, and the choice of non-deliriogenic sedatives and analgesics when needed are all key factors in delirium prevention (Mistraletti et al. 2012).

In recent years, the English National Clinical Guideline Centre (www.nice.org.uk/guidance/CG103) has issued guidelines that revised the most significant studies, conducted in the hospital settings, concerning the efficacy of a multidimensional approach for delirium prevention. International recommendations include the routine evaluation of the main risk factors for delirium (age > 65 years, dementia, hip fracture, and high-risk clinical conditions), in an attempt to identify, beginning at the time of admission to hospital, the most fragile patients, who require the maximum preventive efforts. The following is a list of possible interventions:

- Involve relatives in neurological monitoring to increase the number of controls.
- Program specific meetings for the handover between staff members.
- Organize training courses for operators about validated delirium monitoring tools. Provide continuous visual and auditory media used at home:
  - Place wall clocks, wristwatches, and possibly calendars.
  - Call patients by name.
  - Encourage the placement of pictures or family photographs in the room.
  - Orient the patient's bed so she/he can perceive the alternation of daylight/darkness.
  - Schedule informational interviews with medical personnel concerning diagnostic and therapeutic measures.
- Allow newspaper reading.
- Relaxation interventions.
- Promote nocturnal sleep (silence, vibrating alarms, darkness; avoid nursing procedures whenever possible), discourage daytime sleep, and supplement with melatonin.
- Clinical management interventions.
- Promptly correct hypoxia, hypo/hypertension, anemia, and cardiac arrhythmias.
- Ensure adequate enteral hydration.
- Ensure intake of an adequate amount of calories, trace elements, and vitamins, preferably through the enteral route.
- Encourage the use of dentures whenever possible.
- Facilitate intestinal transit and evacuation.
- Suspend unnecessary drug treatments, especially neuroactive drugs.
- Provide activity rehabilitation/mobilization.
- Provide venous thrombosis prophylaxis.
- Use physical restraints only if strictly necessary.
- Minimize the use of invasive tools (urinary catheter, intravenous infusion lines, and nasogastric tube).
- The use of a flowchart can provide an opportunity to address the problem with an easier-to-handle, step-by-step approach.

Along these lines, physicians and nurses are invited to consider and correct all those factors (i.e., organic and metabolic causes, presence of invasive tools, pain, etc.) that could contribute to delirium development before administering any neuroactive drug (Mistraletti et al. 2012).

Multidisciplinary intervention program including education, guidance, and a changed caring organization reduces the duration of delirium, shortens the length of the hospital stay, and reduces the mortality rate during hospitalization for delirious patients (Lundström et al. 2005). Limitations notwithstanding, the evidence suggests that a broad spectrum of systematic interventions (education, support, reorientation, anxiety reduction, preoperative medical assessment) may be modestly effective in preventing delirium among middle-aged and elderly surgical patients; the median rate of reduction was 13%; interventions by nurses alone were as effective as interventions involving physicians (Cole 1999; Lundström et al. 2005) (see Table 9.1). Pain management eliminate the occurrence of delirium in a frail elderly surgical population (Barr et al. 2013). Nurses should carefully assess pain management in their older patients. Effective pain management reduces the risk for delirium and that nurses should implement effective individualized pain management strategies with clients at risk for or experiencing delirium (Schreier 2010). If using a PCA pump, the older patient's ability to manage the pump should be reassessed often. If a patient is admitted with risk factors for development of delirium, unmanaged pain might be the additional factor that precipitates delirium (Robinson et al. 2008). Proactive geriatric consultation could significantly reduce the incidence of delirium in patients after hip fracture, particularly the incidence of severe delirium. Nurse-led interdisciplinary delirium intervention programs have a positive effect on the incidence and course (severity and duration) of delirium, cognitive functioning, functional rehabilitation, mortality, and length of stay in older hip fracture patients (Inouye et al. 1999; Marcantonio et al. 2003) (see Table 9.2).

**Table 9.1** Recommendations for the prevention of delirium (Michaud et al. 2007)

| General recommendations | Specific recommendations |
|---|---|
| Detect and treat cognitive impairment | Routine screening of cognitive functions and delirium, whenever possible, using standardized instruments (e.g., MMSE or BOMC on admission and CAM during hospital stay)<br>Cognitively stimulating activities adapted to the patient |
| Favor high-quality sleep | Nonpharmacological sleep promotion<br>Noise reduction; use of low-level lighting; avoidance of constant lighting<br>Maintenance of a normal sleep-wake cycle |
| Minimize drug side effects | Limitation of the total number of drugs<br>Avoidance or cautious use of the following medications<br>• Psychotropics, especially hypnosedatives and benzodiazepines<br>• Anticholinergic drugs<br>• Opioids |
| Prevent/correct electrolytic disturbances and dehydration | Stimulation of adequate hydration; use of fluid balance charts<br>Biochemical screening; early management of electrolyte disturbances<br>Hypodermoclysis if oral intake is inadequate |
| Improve communication and orientation | Regular verbal communication; use of short sentences; frequent information on place, reason for hospitalization, and daily activities; whenever possible, involvement of patient in the process of care; information and reassurance about medical procedures<br>On-time Q clocks and calendars; familiar artifacts, whenever possible (i.e., posters); avoidance of ward or room transfers; continuity of care |
| Limit sensory underload or overload | Screening for visual and hearing impairment; provision of visual and hearing aids; adequate lighting; use of night-lights; avoidance of blind rooms (without windows) |
| Involve and inform significant others | Information of proxies regarding delirium; encouragement of visits to the patient and involvement in orientation; nursing and feeding; support of proxies |

(continued)

**Table 9.1** (continued)

| General recommendations | Specific recommendations |
|---|---|
| Avoid malnutrition and vitamin deficiencies | Nutritional support and/or vitamin supplements for high-risk groups (i.e., B vitamins for alcoholic abusers) |
| Prevent or treat withdrawal | If middle-aged adults are at high risk for alcohol withdrawal, prevention with benzodiazepines<br>Clomethiazole for prevention of withdrawal in the elderly<br>Systematic screening for alcohol abuse |
| Do not use physical restraints | Protocol for physical restraints |
| Favor mobilization | Avoidance of immobilization; education regarding hazards of bed rest<br>Limiting the use of catheter and intravenous line; avoidance of the use of Foley catheter<br>Early mobilization protocol; evaluation by physiotherapist, whenever necessary<br>Stimulation of mobility; performance of self-care and daily activities |
| Optimize operative conditions | Adequate analgesia; patient-controlled analgesia, if feasible<br>Prevention of postoperative hypotension/hypoxemia<br>Maintenance of postoperative hematocrit level at >30% |
| Consider interventions on the system | Staff education<br>Development and implementation of guidelines regarding harmful procedures (i.e., physical restraints, medication, unnecessary catheters)<br>Adequate staff allocation<br>Involvement of volunteers and family |

### 9.1.4 Nursing Management of Delirium

The most important action for the management of delirium is the identification and management of the underlying cause. Symptoms are usually reversible when the underlying cause is identified quickly and managed properly, particularly if the cause is hypoglycemia, an infection, an iatrogenic factor, drug toxicity, or an electrolyte imbalance. However, recovery may be slow (days to even weeks), especially in elderly patients. Often the blood tests improve before the patient's brain does. All unnecessary drugs should be stopped. Identifiable disease should be treated, and fluids and nutrients should be given. A patient suspected of alcohol abuse or withdrawal should be given thiamine to ensure absorption. During hospitalization, such patients should be monitored for signs of withdrawal, which can be manifested by autonomic disturbances and worsening confusion and agitation. The environment should be as quiet and calm as possible, preferably with low lighting but not total darkness. Staff and family members should reassure the patient, reinforce orientation, and explain care and proceedings at every opportunity. Additional drugs should be avoided unless they are needed to reverse the underlying condition (Potter and George 2006). Agitation must sometimes be treated symptomatically, especially when it threatens the well-being of the patient, a caregiver, or a staff member. Judicious use of soft restraints can help prevent the patient

**Table 9.2** NICE recommendations for prevention of delirium in at-risk adults (O'Mahony et al. 2011)

| | |
|---|---|
| 1 | Ensure that persons at risk for delirium are cared for by a team of healthcare professionals who are familiar with the person at risk. Avoid moving persons within and between wards or rooms unless absolutely necessary |
| 2 | Give a tailored, multicomponent intervention package. Within 24 h of hospitalization, assess persons at risk for clinical factors contributing to delirium. On the basis of the results of this assessment, provide a multicomponent intervention tailored to the person's individual needs and care setting |
| 3 | The tailored, multicomponent intervention package should be delivered by a multidisciplinary team trained and competent in delirium prevention |
| 4 | Address cognitive impairment or disorientation by providing appropriate lighting and clear signage; ensuring that a clock (consider providing a 24-h clock in the critical care unit) and a calendar are easily visible to the person at risk; talking to the person to reorient them by explaining where they are, who they are, and what your role is; introducing cognitively stimulating activities (e.g., reminiscence); and facilitating regular visits from family and friends |
| 5 | Address dehydration and constipation by ensuring adequate fluid intake to prevent dehydration by encouraging the person to drink—consider offering subcutaneous or intravenous fluids, if necessary, and taking advice when managing fluid balance in persons with comorbid conditions (e.g., heart failure) |
| 6 | Assess for hypoxia and optimize oxygen saturation, if necessary, as clinically appropriate |
| 7 | Address infection by looking for and treating infection, avoiding unnecessary catheterization, and implementing infection-control procedures in line with the NICE clinical guideline on infection control |
| 8 | Address immobility or limited mobility through the following actions: encourage persons to mobilize soon after surgery and walk (provide appropriate walking aids that are accessible at all times) and encourage all persons, including persons who are unable to walk, to carry out active, range-of-motion exercises |
| 9 | Address pain by assessing for pain; looking for nonverbal signs of pain, particularly in persons with communication difficulties (e.g., persons with learning difficulties or dementia or persons on a ventilator or who have a tracheostomy); and initiating and reviewing appropriate pain management in any person in whom pain is identified or suspected |
| 10 | Carry out a medication review for persons receiving several drugs, taking into account both the type and the number of medications |
| 11 | Address poor nutrition by following the advice given in the nutrition support in adults section in the NICE clinical guideline 32 (14) and ensuring that dentures fit properly in persons who have them |
| 12 | Address sensory impairment by resolving any reversible cause of the impairment, such as impacted ear wax, and ensuring hearing and visual aids are available to and used by persons who need them and check that such aids are in good working order |
| 13 | Promote good sleep patterns and sleep hygiene by avoiding nursing or medical procedures during sleeping hours, if possible, scheduling medication rounds to avoid disturbing sleep, and reducing noise to a minimum during sleep periods |

from pulling out intravenous and other lines. Restraints should be applied by someone trained or experienced in their use, released at times to prevent injury, and discontinued as soon as possible. The main symptoms that may require pharmacologic treatment are psychosis and insomnia (Packard 2001). The patient should be nursed in a good sensory environment and with a reality orientation approach and with involvement of the multidisciplinary team (McCusker et al. 2001) (see Table 9.3).

**Table 9.3** Steps in the prevention, diagnosis, and management of delirium (Potter and George 2006)

| | |
|---|---|
| *Step 1*<br>Identify all older patients (over 65 years) with cognitive impairment using the AMT or MMSE on admission | |
| *Step 2*<br>Consider delirium in all patients with cognitive impairment and at high risk (severe illness, dementia, fractured neck of femur, visual and hearing impairment). Use the CAM screening instrument | |
| *Step 3*<br>Identify the cause of delirium if present from the history—obtained from relatives/carers—examination, and investigations. Treat underlying cause or causes—commonly drugs or drug withdrawal, infection, electrolyte disturbance, dehydration, or constipation | |
| *Step 4*<br>In patients with delirium *and* patients at high risk of delirium | |
| *Do*<br>• Provide environmental and personal orientation<br>• Ensure continuity of care<br>• Encourage mobility<br>• Reduce medication but ensure adequate analgesia<br>• Ensure hearing aids and spectacles are available and in good working order<br>• Avoid constipation<br>• Maintain a good sleep pattern<br>• Maintain good fluid intake<br>• Involve relatives and carers (carers leaflet)<br>• Avoid complications (immobility, malnutrition, pressure sores, oversedation, falls, incontinence)<br>• Liaise with old age psychiatry service | *Do not*<br>• Catheterize<br>• Use restraint<br>• Sedate routinely<br>• Argue with the patient |
| *Step 5*<br>If sedation has to be used, use one drug only starting at the lowest possible dose (haloperidol 0.5 mg currently recommended) and increasing in increments, if necessary, after an interval of 2 h | |
| *Step 6*<br>Ensure a safe discharge and consider follow-up with old age psychiatry team<br>Provide family/carer education and support | |

*AMT* abbreviated mental test, *CAM* Confusion Assessment Method, *MMSE* Mini-Mental State Examination

## References

Barr J, Fraser GL, Puntillo K, Ely EW, Gélinas C, Dasta JF et al (2013) Clinical practice guidelines for the management of pain, agitation, and delirium in adult patients in the intensive care unit. Crit Care Med 41(1):263–306. https://doi.org/10.1097/CCM.0b013e3182783b72

Bergeron N, Dubois MJ, Dumont M, Dial S, Skrobik Y (2001) Intensive care delirium screening checklist: evaluation of a new screening tool. Intensive Care Med 27(5):859–864. https://doi.org/10.1007/s001340100909

Chan D, Brennan NJ (1999) Delirium: making the diagnosis, improving the prognosis. Geriatrics 54(3):39–42. http://cat.inist.fr/?aModele=afficheN&cpsidt=9972467

Cole MG (1999) Delirium: effectiveness of systematic interventions. Dement Geriatr Cogn Disord 10(5):406–411. https://doi.org/10.1159/000017179

Csokasy J (1999) Assessment of acute confusion: use of the NEECHAM Confusion Scale. Appl Nurs Res 12(1):51–55

Ely EW, Inouye SK, Bernand GR, Gordon S, Francis J, May L et al (2001) Delirium in mechanically ventilated patients: validity and reliability of the confusion assessment method for the intensive care unit (CAM-ICU). J Am Med Assoc 286(21):2703–2710. http://cat.inist.fr/?aModele=afficheN&cpsidt=13531387

Eden BM, Foreman MD (1996) Problems associated with underrecognition of delirium in critical care: A case study. Heart & Lung: The Journal of Acute and Critical Care 25(5):388–400. https://doi.org/10.1016/S0147-9563(96)80082-3

Flaherty JH, Rudolph J, Shay K, Kamholz B, Boockvar KS, Shaughnessy M et al (2007) Delirium is a serious and under-recognized problem: why assessment of mental status should be the sixth vital sign. J Am Med Dir Assoc 8(5):273–275. https://doi.org/10.1016/j.jamda.2007.03.006

Fong TG, Jones RN, Marcantonio ER, Tommet D, Gross AL, Habtemariam D et al (2012) Adverse outcomes after hospitalization and delirium in persons with Alzheimer disease. Ann Intern Med 156(12):848–856

Gaudreau J-D, Gagnon P, Harel F, Tremblay A, Roy M-A (2005) Fast, systematic, and continuous delirium assessment in hospitalized patients: the nursing delirium screening scale. J Pain Symptom Manag 29(4):368–375. https://doi.org/10.1016/j.jpainsymman.2004.07.009

Inouye SK, Bogardus ST, Charpentier PA, Leo-Summers L, Acampora D, Holford TR, Cooney LM (1999) A multicomponent intervention to prevent delirium in hospitalized older patients. N Engl J Med 340(9):669–676. https://doi.org/10.1056/NEJM199903043400901

Kakuma R, Galbaud du Fort G, Arsenault L, Perrault A, Platt RW, Monette J et al (2003) Delirium in older emergency department patients discharged home: effect on survival. J Am Geriatr Soc 51(4):443–450. https://doi.org/10.1046/j.1532-5415.2003.51151.x

Leslie DL, Marcantonio ER, Zhang Y, Leo-Summers L, Inouye SK (2008) One-year health care costs associated with delirium in the elderly population. Arch Intern Med. 168(1):27–32. https://doi.org/10.1001/archinternmed.2007.4

Luetz A, Heymann A, Radtke FM, Chenitir C, Neuhaus U, Nachtigall I et al (2010) Different assessment tools for intensive care unit delirium: which score to use? Crit Care Med 38(2):409–418. https://doi.org/10.1097/CCM.0b013e3181e0af7c

Lundström M, Edlund A, Karlsson S, Brännström B, Bucht G, Gustafson Y (2005) A multifactorial intervention program reduces the duration of delirium, length of hospitalization, and mortality in delirious patients. J Am Geriatr Soc 53(4):622–628. https://doi.org/10.1111/j.1532-5415.2005.53210.x

Marcantonio ER, Simon SE, Bergmann MA, Jones RN, Murphy KM, Morris JN (2003) Delirium symptoms in post-acute care: prevalent, persistent, and associated with poor functional recovery. J Am Geriatr Soc 51(1):4–9

McCusker J, Cole M, Abrahamowicz M, Han L, Podoba JE, Ramman-Haddad L (2001) Environmental risk factors for delirium in hospitalized older people. J Am Geriatr Soc 49(10):1327–1334. http://doi.org/49260 [pii]

McNicoll L, Pisani MA, Zhang Y, Ely EW, Siegel MD, Inouye SK (2003) Delirium in the intensive care unit: occurrence and clinical course in older patients. J Am Geriatr Soc 51(5):591–598. https://doi.org/10.1034/j.1600-0579.2003.00201.x

Michaud L, Büla C, Berney A, Camus V, Voellinger R, Stiefel F, Burnand B (2007) Delirium: guidelines for general hospitals. J Psychosom Res 62(3):371–383. https://doi.org/10.1016/j.jpsychores.2006.10.004

Milisen K, Lemiengre J, Braes T, Foreman MD (2005) Multicomponent intervention strategies for managing delirium in hospitalized older people: systematic review. J Adv Nurs 52(1):79–90

Mistraletti G, Pelosi P, Mantovani ES, Berardino M, Gregoretti C (2012) Delirium: clinical approach and prevention. Best Pract Res Clin Anaesthesiol 26(3):311–326. https://doi.org/10.1016/j.bpa.2012.07.001

Neelon VJ, Champagne MT, Carlson JR, Funk SG (1996) The NEECHAM Confusion Scale: construction, validation, and clinical testing. Appl Nurs Res 45(6):324–330. http://cat.inist.fr/?aModele=afficheN&cpsidt=10619303

O'Mahony R, Murthy L, Akunne A, Young J (2011) Synopsis of the National Institute for Health and Clinical Excellence guideline for prevention of delirium. Ann Intern Med 154:746–751

Otter H, Martin J, Basell K, von Heymann C, Hein OV, Böllert P et al (2005) Specialized neurocritical care, severity grade, and outcome of patients with aneurysmal subarachnoid hemorrhage. Neurocrit Care 5(2):150–158. https://doi.org/10.1385/Neurocrit

Ouimet S, Kavanagh BP, Gottfried SB, Skrobik Y (2007) Incidence, risk factors and consequences of ICU delirium. Intensive Care Med 33(1):66–73. https://doi.org/10.1007/s00134-006-0399-8

Packard RC (2001) Delirium. Neurologist 7(6):327–340

Potter J, George J (2006) The prevention, diagnosis and management of delirium in older people: concise guidelines. Clin Med (Lond) 6(3):303–308

Rigney TS (2006) Delirium in the hospitalized elder and recommendations for practice. Geriatr Nurs 27(3):151–157. https://doi.org/10.1016/j.gerinurse.2006.03.014

Robinson S, Vollmer C, Jirka H, Rich C, Midiri C, Bisby D (2008) Aging and delirium: too much or too little pain medication? Pain Manag Nurs 9(2):66–72. https://doi.org/10.1016/j.pmn.2007.12.002

Salluh JI, Soares M, Teles JM, Ceraso D, Raimondi N, Nava VS et al (2010) Delirium epidemiology in critical care (DECCA): an international study. Crit Care 14(6):1–7. https://doi.org/10.1186/cc9333

Schreier AM (2010) Nursing care, delirium, and pain management for the hospitalized older adult. Pain Manag Nurs 11(3):177–185. https://doi.org/10.1016/j.pmn.2009.07.002

Sloss EM, Solomon DH, Shekelle PG, Young RT, Saliba D, MacLean CH et al (2000) Selecting target conditions for quality of care improvement in vulnerable older adults. J Am Geriatr Soc 48(4):363–369

Steis MR, Fick DM (2007) Are nurses recognizing delirium? A systematic delirium? J Gerontol Nurs 34(9):40–48

Van den Boogaard M, Pickkers P, van der Hoeven H, Roodbol G, van Achterberg T, Schoonhoven L (2009) Implementation of a delirium assessment tool in the ICU can influence haloperidol use. Crit Care 13(4):1–7. https://doi.org/10.1186/cc7991

# Delirium Prevention: Update on Multidisciplinary, Non-drug Prevention of Delirium Among Hospitalized Elderly

10

Miriam B. Rodin and Joseph H. Flaherty

## 10.1 Introduction

Delirium is a common complication of hospitalized elderly (Inouye et al. 2014). The risk factors for delirium are well understood by hospital care providers (Lee et al. 2013; Cohen and Klein 1958). The focus here will be on non-pharmacological interventions to prevent delirium in non-ICU medical patients for the following reasons: First, the largest patient population is in the general medical wards. Second, the complexity of multicomponent interventions (MCIs) makes them hard to measure since there are many moving parts and disciplines that are not focused on individual clinicians and which vary somewhat from study to study. Lastly, the data from different meta-analyses are not in agreement. Thus, the purpose of this paper is to help clinicians to conceptualize delirium based on risk factors for delirium and the basic principles of MCIs in a way that helps them as an individual clinician "do" their part of the MCI within a supportive hospital system (Bergmann 2005; Clegg et al. 2014).

## 10.2 Trials of Non-pharmacological Interventions to Prevent Delirium

The 2016 update of the 2007 Cochrane review includes a plethora of new studies assessing the efficacy of pharmacologic treatment and prevention of delirium mostly targeted at critically ill ICU, trauma, and surgery patients (Siddiqui et al. 2007). The review included five additional high-quality RCTs. The reviewers concluded that these seven studies in total provided "moderate quality" evidence for clinically significant effectiveness of multicomponent non-pharmacological interventions (MCI)

M.B. Rodin, M.D., Ph.D. (✉) • J.H. Flaherty, M.D.
Division of Geriatric Medicine, Department of Internal Medicine, St. Louis School of Medicine, St. Louis, MO, USA


A.T. Isik, G.T. Grossberg (eds.), *Delirium in Elderly Patients*,
https://doi.org/10.1007/978-3-319-65239-9_10

to prevent delirium among the pooled sample of nearly 2000 mostly elderly non-ICU hospital inpatients shown in Table 10.1 (Abizanda et al. 2011; Bonaventura and Zanotti 2007; Hempenius et al. 2013; Jeffs et al. 2013; Lundstrom et al. 2007; Marcantonio et al. 2001; Martinez et al. 2012). The effect sizes of pooled studies of medical patients were slightly larger than for a separate analysis of 22 orthogeriatric hip fracture studies summarized in Table 10.2 (Siddiqui et al. 2007). Of note, the studies excluded dementia patients in whom the overwhelming risk for delirium could wash out more modest gains among cognitively intact patients.

A separate meta-analysis by Hshieh et al. included nonrandomized studies (NRT) if there was a control (synchronous or historical) or matched comparison group and

**Table 10.1** Summary of non-pharmacological CTs

| First author | Year | *N*= | Interventions | Outcomes |
|---|---|---|---|---|
| A. *RCTs selected for Cochrane analysis 9* | | | | |
| Abizanda et al. (2011) | 2011 | | 1, 3, 7, 10 | 1, 7, 13 |
| Bonaventura and Zanotti (2007) | 2007 | | 3, 4, 5, 6, 8 | 1, 6, 8 |
| | | | 10, 11 | |
| Hempenius et al. (2013) | 2013 | | 1, 2, 4, 5, 8 | 1, 2, 4, 5, 10 |
| | | | 9, 10, 11, 13 | 14 |
| | | | 16, 17, 18, 19 | |
| Jeffs et al.* (2013) | 2013 | | 4, 10 | 1, 2, 3, 5, 6 |
| Lundstrom et al.* (2007) | 2006 | | 1, 2, 3, 8, 9 | 1, 3, 4, 5, 6, 9 |
| | | | 10, 11, 12, 13 | 11, 12 |
| | | | 14, 16, 19 | |
| Marcantonio et al. (2001) | 2001 | | 1 | 1, 2, 3, 5, 6, 11, 13 |
| Martinez et al.* (2012) | 2012 | | 3, 4, 5, 6 | 1, 3, 4, 6 |
| B. *Studies included in JAMA analysis*17* | | | | |
| Andro et al. (2012) | 2012 | 256 | 4, 5, 8, 10 | 1 |
| Babine et al. (2013) | 2013 | 516 | 4, 5, 8, 10, 11 | 4 |
| Bo et al. (2009) | 2009 | 252 | 4, 8, 10, 11 | 1, 6 |
| Bogardus et al. (2003) | 2003 | 705 | 4, 5, 8, 10, 11 | 5 |
| Caplan and Harper (2007) | 2007 | 37 | 4, 5, 8 | 1, 4, 5, 6, 7, 8 |
| Chen et al.** (2011) | 2011 | 179 | 4, 10 | 1, 6, 7, 8 |
| Holt et al. (2013) | 2013 | 362 | 4, 5, 8, 10 | 1, 5, 6 |
| Inouye et al. (1999) | 1999 | 852 | 4, 5, 8, 10, 11 | 1, 6, 7, 8 |
| Kratz (2008) | 2008 | 137 | 4, 5, 8, 10, 11 | 1 |
| Stenvall et al.** (2007) | 2007 | 199 | 5, 10, 11 | 4, 6 |
| Vidan et al. (2009) | 2009 | 542 | 4, 5, 8, 10, 11 | 1, 6, 7 |

Interventions: 1. Individual care plan, 2. Check lists, protocols, 3. Staff education, 4. Reorientation, 5. Sensory deprivation, 6. Familiar objects, 7. Cognitive stimulation, 8. Nutrition, hydration, 9. Search for infection, 10. Mobilization, 11. Sleep hygiene, 12. Multidisciplinary team care, 13. CGA, 14. Oxygenation, 15. Electrolytes, 16. Pain, 17. Polypharmacy, medication review, 18. Mood, 19. Bowel and bladder

Outcomes reported: 1. Delirium incidence, 2. Delirium severity, 3. Delirium duration, 4. Falls, 5. DC to LTC/NH, 6. LOS, 7. Decreased ADL, 8. Decreased cognition, 9. Pressure ulcers, 10. Mental health, 11. Inpatient mortality, 12. 2-month mortality, 13. Medical complications, 14. Surgical complications

* Means this citation was included in the Cochrane (Siddiqui) meta-analysis

** Means this study was included in both the Cochrane (Siddiqui) and the JAMA (Hsieh) meta-analyses

**Table 10.2** Meta-analysis of clinical trials of multicomponent interventions to prevent delirium in hospitalized elderly medical patients

| | Cochrane 2016 review of RCTs $N = 7$[a] | | | | JAMA 2015 review of NRTs $N = 11$[b] | | | |
|---|---|---|---|---|---|---|---|---|
| Outcomes | # Studies | # Subjects | RR | CI | # Studies | # Subjects | RR | CI |
| **Incident delirium** | **4** | **1365** | **0.63** | **0.43, 0.92**[c] | **11** | **2022** | **0.47** | **0.38, 0.58**[c] |
| LOS | 3 | 1335 | 0.04 | −0.44, 0.52 | 10 | 1820 | −0.16 | −0.97, 0.64 |
| Cognitive decline | 1 | 60 | 9.10 | 7.20, 11.00[c] | 3 | 896 | 0.97 | −0.46,2.41 |
| **Falls** | **1** | **287** | **0.11** | **0.01, 2.03** | **4** | **519** | **0.38** | **0.25, 0.60**[c] |
| ADL decline | 1 | 341 | 1.15 | 0.91, 1.47 | 4 | 524 | 0.57 | −0.03, 1.18 |
| Institutionalization | 1 | 648 | 0.96 | 0.88, 1.06 | 4 | 619 | 0.95 | 0.71, 1.26 |
| Citations | | | | | | | | |

[a]RCTs: Abizanda, Bonaventura, Hempenius, Jeffs, Lundstrom, Marcantonio, Martinez
[b]NRT: Bo, Caplan, Chen, Holt, Inouye, Jeffs, Martinez, Lundstrom, Vidan
[c]Statistically significant

the studies met other standard criteria of quality (Hshieh et al. 2015). Three of the Cochrane randomized studies were included among the 14 chosen for meta-analysis (Jeffs et al. 2013; Lundstrom et al. 2007; Martinez et al. 2012; Andro et al. 2012; Babine et al. 2013; Bo et al. 2009; Bogardus et al. 2003; Caplan and Harper 2007; Chen et al. 2011; Holt et al. 2013; Inouye et al. 1999). Table 10.1 lists the studies, the sample sizes, and the non-pharmacological multicomponent interventions (MCI) that were implemented and which outcome measures were reported for these two meta-analyses.

Table 10.2 shows the shared end points reported by RCTs and NRTs. All studies reported incidence of delirium, but they used different protocols for surveillance, as well as different validated assessment tools. The RCTs reported a pooled RR 0.69 (0.59–0.81) for incident delirium for MCI (Siddiqui et al. 2007). The NRTs reported a pooled RR 0.47 (0.38–0.58) reduction in incidence of delirium (Hshieh et al. 2015). Four RCTs considered the duration of delirium, and two recorded severity. Six of seven RCTs reported hospital length of stay, RR 0.01 (−0.48, 0.51). Five of 11 NRTs reported similar results, RR −0.16 (−0.97, 0.64). Three RCTs and no NRTs reported hospital mortality. Four RCTs and four NRTs reported changes in measures of functional status at discharge or at some later date. The confidence intervals indicated no statistical significance in the pooled analyses for reduction in functional impairment or, depending on the study, the degree of functional impairment or improvement at discharge.

Table 10.3 summarizes the findings of both analyses for outcomes of MCI. For comparison of effect sizes, the pooled results of pharmacological trials to prevent delirium among non-ICU medical patients were RR 0.73 (0.33, 1.59) among 916 patients treated with prophylactic antipsychotics (olanzapine and haloperidol) and RR 0.68 (0.17, 2.62) among 113 patients treated prophylactically with donepezil (Siddiqui et al. 2007). These results suggest that MCI may be as or more effective than drug prophylaxis in preventing delirium among medical inpatients.

Multicomponent non-pharmacological interventions can vary markedly from one another, and so pooling them to assess effectiveness as a general approach hides important differences among them. The analysts attempt to control for unmeasurable variability by using appropriate statistical adjustments. For example, LOS determinations were analyzed using random effects models to adjust for

**Table 10.3** Meta-analysis of outcomes of multicomponent interventions (Cochrane review)

| Outcome measure | Pooled *N*= | RR | CI |
|---|---|---|---|
| QOL: mental health | 246 | 0.88 | 0.64, 1.20[a] |
| UTI incident | 260 | 1.20 | 0.45, 3.20 |
| Cardiovascular event | 260 | 1.13 | 0.78, 1.65 |
| 12-month mortality | 199 | 0.85 | 0.46, 1 .56[a] |
| Inpatient mortality | 859 | 0.90 | 0.56, 1.43[a] |
| Pressure ulcers | 457 | 0.48 | 0.26, 0.89 |
| Falls | 746 | 0.57 | 0.16, 2.01 |
| Depression | 149 | 0.70 | −0.44, 1.84[a] |
| Return to indep living | 1116 | 0.95 | 0.85, 1.06[a] |
| ADL performance | 341 | 1.15 | 0.91, 1.47[a] |
| Cognitive status | 30 | 9.10 | 7.20, 11.00[a] |

[a]Attributable to severity of illness, frailty, and multimorbidity and unlikely to be affected by brief inpatient intervention

unmeasured and uncontrollable institutional variability in discharging practices (Siddiqui et al. 2007; Hshieh et al. 2015). It may be that each component within a bundled intervention might affect different specific outcomes. Alternatively it is difficult to determine whether bundled interventions are additive, multiplicative, or just redundant. It is methodologically almost impossible to tease out what component in a bundle made a difference vs. the entirety of the approach to care.

The components of non-pharmacological delirium prevention are directed to modifying known risk factors for delirium. The NICE working group proposed a streamlined list of risk factors: age over 65 years, cognitive impairment, hip fracture, and severe illness (Young et al. 2010). None of these risk factors can be modified. Other lists of risk factors include mixtures of patient, disease, and environmental factors. Risk factors for delirium include age; dementia; severity of illness; polypharmacy especially use of sedatives, hypnotics, and opiates; immobility as a manifestation of frailty; immobility due to the illness; and immobilization due to treatment. De facto restraints on movement include hospital equipment designed for maximization of caregiver efficiency such as electric adjustable height beds with rails, tables and portable equipment on wheels, and multiple non-integrated auditory alarms and sleep deprivation due to hospital routines. In the context of patient weakness, pain, sleep deprivation, and preexisting sensory deficits, environmental factors have been treated as fixed and not as risk factors to be ameliorated. However, this may be changing (Wong et al. 2014). Figure 10.1 organizes risk factors by whether they are intrinsic to the patient (host), the disease or injury that brought the patient to the hospital (agent), and the hospital environment. Arrows show possible pathways of host, agent, and environment feedback that result in delirium.

The classical epidemiological triangle presumes that disease is the result of a susceptible host encountering a virulent agent due to an environment or vector that brings them into contact. Prevention can happen at any accessible link in the system. By dividing the MCI model this way, it allows the clinician to conceptualize the items in the boxes as either "intrinsic" (host and agent) or "extrinsic" (hospital).

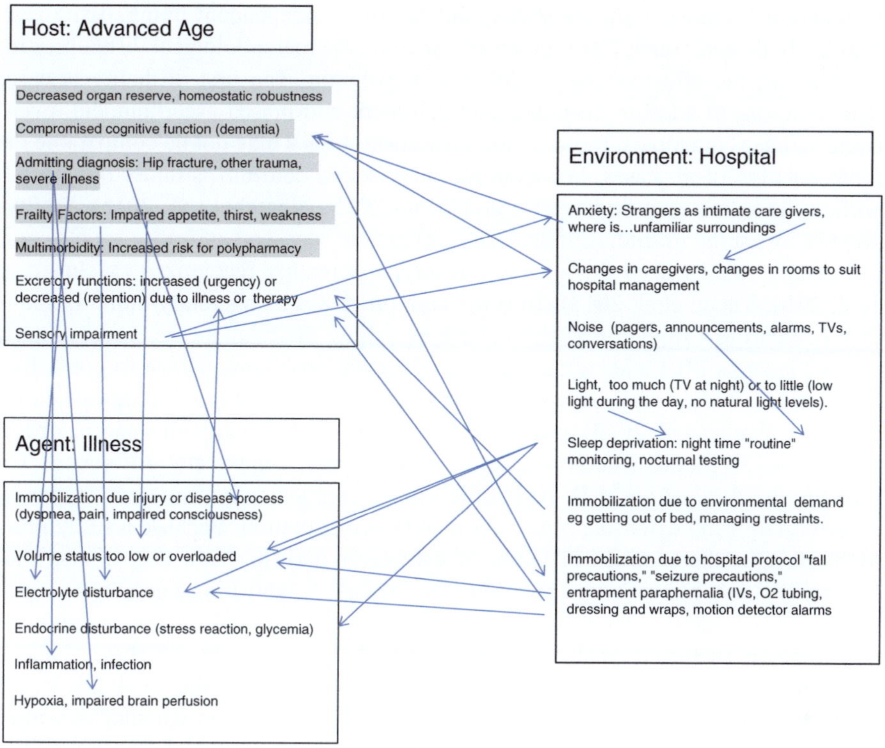


**Fig. 10.1** Interaction of host, agent and environment in the etiology of hospital-acquired delirium in elderly medical inpatients

Rather than approach delirium as this overwhelming "multifactorial" complex situation, the clinicians can first focus on individual items as they can control. For example, a clinician can make sure that all the intrinsic items in "agent" are treated optimally. Next, the clinician can identify "extrinsic" items in "hospital" and then work with nursing staff and others to alleviate or fix these. By doing this, we can deconstruct delirium to identify what we can control and what we cannot. Host characteristics such as age, frailty, and cognitive impairment cannot be modified in the context of an acute hospitalization but drugs, changes in rooming and staffing, and intrusive monitoring can be (Otremba et al. 2016). Sensory deficits can be ameliorated by using hearing and visual aids. We can treat the illness and we can change the environment.

## 10.3 Why Are We Not Convinced?

The RCTs have been reasonably consistent in showing about a 30% reduction in incidence of delirium. But delirium researchers have confessed a certain amount of despair that this has not translated into improved longer-term outcomes with regard to functional status, cognitive status, and return to independent living. Teale and Young (Teale and Young 2015) concisely detailed the methodological difficulties in establishing the effectiveness of delirium prevention. The first difficulty is case identification. In addition to under ascertainment and biased ascertainment, even using standard diagnostic tools, single institution studies may not be comparable or representative of all cases. For example, hypoactive delirium is under diagnosed without intensive case finding (De and Wand 2015; Albrecht et al. 2015). Frailty must be measured in studies of delirium prevention. Measures of frailty are also not universally standardized though the phenotype is readily recognized (Malmstron et al. 2014; Theou et al. 2013). To study care processes is inherently more difficult than comparing a single intervention such as a drug. Studying a care process intervention such as MCI adds additional measurement problems. A case in point, the hip fracture studies vary by whether all hip fracture patients are geographically cohorted (Watne et al. 2014) or roomed throughout the hospital with standing order sets and MDT rounds (SteelFisher et al. 2013). Does it make any difference? To measure the dose of an MCI intervention in a geographically scattered sample is difficult, requiring extensive observation and documentation. Because a study protocol changes the routines of shifts of caregivers and therefore also affects the supervisors' job, maintaining consistency is difficult. Establishing a geographic unit is probably essential to program delivery, but the organizational barriers are high. A recent review by Inouye et al. into failures of HELP sites identified high-level leadership as the key to program survival and effectiveness (SteelFisher et al. 2013).

As shown in Table 10.3, well-done studies that investigated whether delirium prevention in the hospital improves outcomes weeks and months later report disappointing results, but that should not be taken on face value. Some delirium resolves promptly, some resolves never in life. How this relates to one episode of hospital care is not direct or obvious. Orthogeriatric units have been more widely adopted in Europe than in the USA. These units cohort elderly hip fracture patients for more consistent delivery of MCI. Table 10.4 summarizes the findings reported for the orthogeriatric units (Siddiqui et al. 2007). Both Tables 10.3 and 10.4 are inconclusive. The host and agent factors present from the start of care may not be easily changed and may be what explains post-hospital outcomes regardless of medical intervention. The further out from an acute illness, the more likely other factors are driving the outcomes. As argued by Teale and Young (Teale and Young 2015), long-term outcomes are more likely to be due to the disease and the underlying and unmeasured frailty of the host. The only study that specifically examined frailty as a risk factor, the original report on the HELP intervention in 1999, reported all of the substantial benefit in reduced incidence, and improved functional outcome was seen among the non-frail subjects (Bogardus et al. 2003).

Delirium is a sentinel event in the natural history of frailty. We presently have no effective interventions to reverse established frailty, so studies of delirium should upfront stratify patients using a validated assessment of premorbid frailty. There are numbers of assessment tools that have been validated and tested against one another (Malmstron et al. 2014; Theou et al. 2013). Frailty assessments can be completed with patients or by proxy in a few minutes. Looking again at Fig. 10.1, the known

**Table 10.4** Outcomes of 22 geriatric units for the care of surgical/hip fracture patients

| Outcome | RR | Confidence intervals |
|---|---|---|
| Delirium incidence | 0.98 | 0.79–1.22 |
| Delirium severity | 1.50 | −1.00–4.00 |
| Delirium duration | −1.00 | −2.04–0.04 |
| **Hospital LOS** | **3.00** | **1.94–4.06** |
| Adverse events | 0.96 | 0.76–1.23 |
| Pressure ulcers | 0.38 | −6.10–1.41 |
| Falls | 1.30 | 0.61–2.77 |
| Inpatient mortality | 0.56 | 0.21–1.47 |
| Care Home at 4 months | 1.06 | 0.58–1.91 |
| Care Home at 12 months | 0.86 | 0.47–1.59 |
| ADL decline at 4 months | 1.00 | −0.70–2.70 |
| New dementia year | 2.26 | 0.60–8.49 |

Abstracted from Siddiqui et al. 2016

risk factors for delirium are highly prevalent in frail patients even when they are not acutely ill. The essential features of frailty including weakness, falls, fatigue, and poor appetite make hospitals as usual riskier for frail patients. At the same time, hospitals are intensely risk averse. US hospitals do not routinely screen for delirium but they do screen all patients for fall risk (Lindquist and Sendelbach 2007; Corsovini et al. 2009). Since the risk factors are the same, it would seem no more difficult to identify "delirium-risk" patients on admission. Thus, high-risk patients can be preferentially assigned to specialized delirium nursing units, ACE (Acute Care of the Elderly) or GEM (Geriatric Evaluation and Management) units. Low-risk patients can be admitted to the general population and intermediate-risk patients, and the "vulnerable" elderly could be cohorted close to the ACE unit or managed by MCI teams with orders consistent with ACE protocols. This approach has been tried with some success but without the rigorous design required by meta-analytics (Avendano-Cespedes et al. 2016; Gentric et al. 2007; Tay and Chan 2013; Pitkala et al. 2008; Bakker et al. 2014; Flood et al. 2013).

## 10.4 If You Cannot Modify the Host, Modify the Environment

The idea of a specialized acute care of elderly hospital unit has been investigated as a way to bring to bear all findings of delirium studies and fall studies (Ahmed and Pearce 2010; Lafont et al. 2011). The essential character of an ACE that differentiates it from usual acute hospital units is that it superficially resembles a VA GEM rehabilitation unit, an inpatient mental health or other intermediate care unit. The critical components of an ACE unit, however, are that it is targeted to high medical acuity patients, those at highest risk for delirium and for falls. The multidisciplinary teams, usually led by a geriatrician, are not consultants. They are physically present and rounding on a geographically discreet unit of anywhere from 10 to 48 beds. There are formal rounds and the daily processes of care are unit based and nurse led. This has a significant impact on adherence to principles of care and may represent the best shot at maximizing the dose of environmental MDI (Fletcher et al. 2007). For example, the key requirement for early mobilization goes directly against some nurses' training to promote comfort and institutional pressure to enforce a "culture of safety." In a fascinating mixed-method study, Doherty-King and Bowers reported, "For all nurses, acutely ill patients are limited to bed mobility. Once physiologically stable, getting up to a chair or ambulation can be considered" (Doherty-King and Bowers 2010). They conclude that the cultural norm for hospital nurses does not consider mobilization to be part of routine care. Ambulation is considered a safety measure to prevent complications such as DVT and pressure ulcers, a way to monitor progress toward discharge and for compliance with doctors' orders. These investigators found that the best predictor of nurses' decisions about mobilizing patients had to do with unit expectations, the microculture of each nursing unit.

Ahmed et al. reviewed reports of ACE unit outcomes and found increased or neutral initial costs in five RCTs. Some have reported cost savings (Avendano-Cespedes et al. 2016; Flood et al. 2013). Outcomes of LOS and readmission were neutral or better; functional outcomes were neutral or better. These trials did not report on delirium outcomes. However, two (Covinsky et al. 1997; Counsell et al. 2000) of five RCTs reported increased caregiver job satisfaction. Studies with weaker designs have also reported this (Benedict et al. 2006; Palmer 2003; Flaherty et al. 2003). Few studies of ACE units have reported delirium outcomes. Several early studies varied but were generally positive (Flaherty et al. 2003; Allen et al. 2003; Aspelund et al. 2000). More recent studies report variable effect sizes. A study in Spain compared ACE to usual care and reported a parallel group $N = 50$ blinded prospective trial 27% reduction in delirium incidence (Avendano-Cespedes et al. 2016). A Swiss study reported a pre-post design study $N = 739$ with RR reduction of 73% overall and 66% among patients with dementia (Gentric et al. 2007). The underlying rates however were quite low in both groups, so these estimates are likely unstable. Bo et al. (2009) and Vidan et al. (2009) reported NRTs with results as shown in Table 10.2. Treating delirium in designated delirium units may be effective for improved immediate- and short-term results (Tay and Chan 2013; Pitkala et al. 2008). Studies show neutral or decreased cost of delirium care in several different health systems (SteelFisher et al. 2013; Lindquist and Sendelbach 2007; Corsovini et al. 2009; Avendano-Cespedes et al. 2016; Aspelund et al. 2000).

## 10.5 Where from Here?

Because of study design differences among the many published reports, it is difficult to pull out clear lessons, especially those that will be persuasive to hospital managers. Future studies should begin with routine assessment on admission for known delirium risk factors including validated measures of frailty. By correctly classifying hospitalized elderly as fit, vulnerable, or frail, that is, high, moderate, or low risk for delirium outcome, studies would then be able to stratify patients by risk level. This would accomplish two things. First, it would establish whether benefit from intervention is linked to risk that would permit better allocation of patients to designated units in practice. If MCI interventions can be standardized between sites, as was done with the HELP programs, pooled data would be more informative. We routinely risk stratify patients for adverse events in surgery, for tolerance of chemotherapy, for alcohol withdrawal, and for falls. In deciding how to apply these tools, we use published data, the evidence, to calculate patients' risk to benefit ratio of invasive or toxic treatments. Looking again at Fig. 10.1, the hospital environment is an agent of delirium. Redesigning environments and choosing different care protocols for high-, moderate-, and low-risk patients are really a decision about patient-centered vs. hospital-centered care.

Cui bono? If we have carefully conducted trials of stratifying patients on risk for delirium that cohorts high-risk patients in geographically designated ACE units, moderate-risk patients in step-down MCI care, and low-risk patients to the general hospital, we may discover which patients benefit and how much by which model of MCI. The usual metrics of hospital risk reduction can be applied. These include not only delirium but exacerbations of CHF, pneumonia, UTIs, falls, medical complications, LOS, readmissions, and discharges to long-term care. It would also permit tracking the metrics of patient satisfaction, family satisfaction, and staff satisfaction. Several studies have reported increased provider satisfaction (Covinsky et al. 1997; Counsell et al. 2000; Benedict et al. 2006; Palmer 2003; Flaherty et al. 2003) and on family and patient satisfaction with care (Covinsky et al. 1997; Counsell et al. 2000)

Healthcare organizations pay attention to satisfaction metrics (Lee et al. 2013). Healthcare organizations invest in staff development and training, and staff turnover is a metric of how well the management has built morale. Nurse retention depends not only on pay scales and accommodating schedules. Caregivers who feel membership on an expert team may be less likely to leave. Systems can be redesigned to change what is done physically to the patient, changes in the immediate sensory surround of the patient, and reorganizing the chains of communication so that care providers interact differently with each other to distribute care tasks (Tay and Chan 2013; Covinsky et al. 1997; Flaherty et al. 2003). This requires a top-down investment in implementation such as training, education, and sharing management decisions. It requires continuous self-monitoring within the work group. There must be structures for sustaining the culture (Tay and Chan 2013).

Modifying an entire hospital or floor or wing or cluster of beds to reduce the toxicity of a normal hospital floor will have necessarily a different effect than individualizing care that does not change the surround. Elements of environmental redesign include establishing normal diurnal activity and light levels. Noise reduction requires reengineering communication to eliminate overhead announcements, the content of which is mostly distressing. There are established guidelines for acceptable noise levels during the day. It is not just the decibels but also the quality of the sounds that require redesign. Soundproofing can muffle hallway conversation. Redesigning monitoring technology such as motion detectors, vital signs monitors and IV pump alarms would reduce alarm fatigue on the staff and noise pollution for the patients. Airplane style disposable headphones can eliminate the competition between TVs on different stations. By designing accommodations to facilitate direct line of sight observation for nursing staff, the impetus for restraints is reduced. Bundled protocols for mobilization, activities, feeding, and assessments require nurses and other caregivers to remember and change gears on a bed-by-bed basis. It would be difficult if not impossible to deliver each of these interventions to individual patients scattered throughout the hospital. Environmental interventions cannot be as effective on room-by-room basis. There is more likely to be inconsistent adherence which has been shown to be critical to effectiveness (Aspelund et al. 2000). The best known and evaluated program is the HELP, Hospital Elder Life Program. The HELP group has had the ability to implement the program in over 100 different hospitals and has the most extensive experience with how and when MCI works and when it fails. In all cases the key to sustaining delirium prevention programs is buy-in from hospital and nursing leadership and having physician champions visible daily on the floors (Wong et al. 2014).

## 10.6 Summary

This narrative review has drawn heavily on the best and most comprehensive analytic reviews of trials of MCI for delirium prevention and management over the past 25 years. There is cause for hope in that the methodologically strongest studies support a 30% reduction of incident delirium among hospitalized elders. However, there are great disparities in measures, outcomes, and interventions. The improvement in post-hospital outcomes has been more difficult to establish. As geriatricians we see the clustering of syndromes among the same types of patients who have been identified as frail. Frailty is at the core of risk factors for delirium, but we have no ways to reverse it. Using the metaphor of the epidemiologic triangle of host, agent, and environment, we can view the hospital as either the agent or the environment inducing delirium vulnerable elderly. With all the caveats about heterogeneity of studies, redesigned patient care practices and hospital environments appear to be effective in preventing delirium. These measures appear to be at least cost neutral and to improve patient, family, and staff morale. Future studies should stratify patients on delirium risk as a means to admit them to appropriate hospital units. If investigators can agree on a set of assessments and standardize environmental designs, we will have the means to conduct the multicenter trials that are needed to prove or disprove the value of specialized acute care of the elderly.

## References

Abizanda P, Leon M, Dominguez-Martin L et al (2011) Effects of a short-term occupational therapy intervention in an acute geriatric unit. Maturitas 69:273–278

Ahmed NN, Pearce SE (2010) Acute care for the elderly: a literature review. Popul Health Manag 13:219–225

Albrecht JS, Marcantonio ER, Roffey DM, Orwig D, Magaziner J, Terrin M, Carson JL, Barr E, Brown JP, Gentry EG, Gruber-Baldini AL (2015) Functional outcomes in cardiovascular patients undergoing surgical hip fracture repair cognitive ancillary study investigators. Stability

of postoperative delirium psychomotor subtypes in individuals with hip fracture. J Am Geriatr Soc 63:970–976
Allen KR, Hazelett SE, Palmer RR et al (2003) Developing a stroke unit using the acute care for elders intervention and model of care. J Am Geriatr Soc 51:1660–1667
Andro M, Comps E, Estivin S, Gentric A (2012) Prevention of delirium in demented hospitalized patients. Eur J Intern Med 23:124–125
Aspelund K, Gustafson Y, Jacobsson C et al (2000) Geriatric-based vs general wards for older acute medical patients: a randomized comparison of outcomes and use of resources. J Am Geriatr Soc 48:1381–1388
Avendano-Cespedes A, Garcia Cantos N, Gonzalez-Teruel M et al (2016) Pilot study of a preventive multicomponent nurse intervention to reduce the incidence and severity of delirium in hospitalized older adults: MID-Nurse-P. Maturitas 86:86–94
Babine RL, Farrington S, Wierman HR (2013) HELP prevent falls by preventing delirium. Nursing 43:18–21
Bakker FC, Persoon A, Bredie SJH et al (2014) The CareWell in Hospital program to improve the quality of care for frail elderly inpatients: results of a before-after study with focus on surgical patients. Am J Surg 208:735–746
Benedict L, Robinson K, Holder C (2006) Clinical nurse specialist practice within the Acute Care for Elders interdisciplinary team model. Clin Nurse Spec 20:248–251
Bergmann MA (2005) Outcomes of older people admitted to post-acute facilities with delirium. J Am Geriatr Soc 53:963–969
Bo M, Martini M, Ruatta C et al (2009) Geriatric ward hospitalization reduced incidence delirium among older medical inpatients. Am J Geriatr Psychiatry 17:760–768
Bogardus ST, Desai MM, Williams CS et al (2003) The effects of a targeted multicomponent delirium intervention on post discharge outcomes for hospitalized older adults. Am J Med 114:383–390
Bonaventura M, Zanotti R (2007) Effectiveness of "IPD" treatment for delirium prevention in hospitalized elderly: a controlled randomized clinical trial. Prof Inferm 60:230–236
Caplan GA, Harper EL (2007) Recruitment of volunteers to improve vitality in the elderly: the REVIVE study. Intern Med J 37:95–100
Chen CC, Lin MT, Tien YW et al (2011) Modified hospital elder life program effects on abdominal surgery patients. J Am Coll Surg 213:245–252
Clegg A, Siddiqui N, Heaven A et al (2014) Interventions for preventing delirium in older people in institutional long term care. Cochrane Database Syst Rev. (1)CD009537
Cohen S, Klein HK (1958) The delirious patient. Am J Nursing 58:685–687
Corsovini L, Bo M, Aimonino NR et al (2009) Predictors of falls and hospitalization outcomes in elderly patients admitted to an acute geriatric unit. Arch Gerontol Geriatr 49:142–145
Counsell SR, Holder CM, Liebenauer LL et al (2000) Effects of a multicomponent intervention on functional outcomes and process of care in hospitalized older patients. A randomized, controlled trial of Acute Care for Elders (ACE) in a community hospital. J Am Geriatr Soc 48:1572–1581
Covinsky KE, King JT Jr, Quinn LM et al (1997) Do acute care for the elders units increase hospital costs? A cost analysis using the hospital perspective. J Am Geriatr Soc 45:729–734
De J, Wand AP (2015) Delirium screening: a systematic review of delirium screening tools in hospitalized patients. Gerontologist 55:1079–1099
Doherty-King B, Bowers B (2010) How nurses decide to ambulate hospitalized older adults: development of a conceptual model. Gerontologist 51:786–797
Flaherty JH, Tariq SH, Raghavan S et al (2003) A model for managing delirious older inpatients. J Am Geriatr Soc 51:1031–1035
Fletcher K, Hawkes P, Williams-Rosenthal S et al (2007) Using nurse practitioners to implement best practice care for the elderly during hospitalization: the NICHE journey at the University of Virginia Medical Center. Crit Care Clin North Am 19:321–337
Flood KL, MacClennan PA, McGrew D et al (2013) Effects of an acute care for elders unit on costs and 30-day readmissions. JAMA Intern Med 173:981–987

Gentric A, Le Deum P, Estivin S (2007) Prevention du syndrome confusionnel dans un service de medicine interne geriatrique. La Rev Med Interne 28:589–593
Hempenius L, Slaets JPJ, van Asselt D et al (2013) Outcomes of a geriatric iaison intervention to prevent the development of post-operative delirium in frail elderly cancer patients: report on a multicenter, randomized, controlled trial. PLoS One 8:e64834
Holt R, Young J, Heseltine D (2013) Effectiveness of a multi-component intervention to reduce delirium incidence in elderly care wards. Age Ageing 42:721–727
Hshieh TT, Yue JR, Oh E et al (2015) Effectiveness of multicomponent nonpharmacological delirium interventions: a meta-analysis. JAMA Intern Med 175:512–520
Inouye SK, Bogardus ST Jr, Charpentier PA et al (1999) A multicomponent intervention to prevent delirium in hospitalized older patients. N Engl J Med 340:669–676
Inouye SK, Westendorp RG, Saczynski JS (2014) Delirium in elderly people. Lancet 383:911–922
Jeffs KJ, Berlowitz DJ, Grant S et al (2013) An enhanced exercise and cognitive programme does not appear to reduce incident delirium in hospitalized patients: a randomized, controlled trial. BMJ Open 3:e002569
Kratz A (2008) Use of the acute confusion protocol: a research utilization project. J Nurs Care Qual 23:331–337
Lafont C, Gerard S, Voisin T et al (2011) Reducing "iatrogenic disability" in the hospitalized frail elderly. J Nutr Health Aging 15:645–660
Lee EA, Gibbs NE, Fahey L, Whiffen TL (2013) Making hospitals safer for older adults: updating quality metrics by understanding hospital-acquired delirium and its link to falls. Perm J 17:32–36
Lindquist R, Sendelbach SE (2007) Maximizing safety of hospitalized elders. Crit Care Nurs Clin North Am 19:277–284
Lundstrom M, Olofsson B, Stenvall M et al (2007) Postoperative delirium in old patients with femoral neck fracture: a randomized intervention study. Aging Clin Exp Res 19:178–186
Malmstron TK, Miller DK, Morley JE (2014) A comparison of four frailty models. J Am Geriatr Soc 62:721–726
Marcantonio ER, Flacker JM, Wright RJ, Resnick NM (2001) Reducing delirium after hip fracture: a randomized trial. J Am Geriatr Soc 49:516–522
Martinez FT, Tobar C, Beddings CI, Vallejo G (2012) Preventing delirium in an acute hospital using a non-pharmacological intervention. Age Ageing 41:629–634
Otremba I, Wilczynski K, Szewieczek J (2016) Delirium in the geriatric unit: proton-pump inhibitors and other risk factors. Clin Interv Aging 11:397–405
Palmer R (2003) Acute care for elders: practical considerations for optimizing health outcomes. Dis Manag Health Outcomes 11:507–517
Pitkala KH, Laurila JV, Standberg TE et al (2008) Multicomponent geriatric intervention for elderly inpatients with delirium: effects on costs and health-related quality of life. J Gerontol Med Sci 63A:56–61
Siddiqui N, Harrison JK, Clegg A et al (2007) Interventions for preventing delirium in hospitalized non-ICU patients (Review) Update of Cochrane Database of Systematic Reviews. (2) CD005563. PMID 17443600, (2016)
SteelFisher GK, Martin LA, Dowal SL, Inouye SK (2013) Learning from the closure of clinical programs: a case series from the Hospital Elder Life Program. J Am Geriatr Soc 61:994–1004
Stenvall M, Olofsson B, Lundstrom M et al (2007) A multidisciplinary, multifactorial intervention program reduces postoperative falls and injuries after femoral neck fracture. Osteoporos Int 18:167–175
Tay LBG, Chan MPC (2013) Functional improvement in hospitalized older adults is independent of dementia diagnosis: experience of a specialized delirium management unit. J Hosp Med 8:321–327
Teale E, Young J (2015) Multicomponent delirium prevention: not as effective as NICE suggests? Age Ageing 44:915–917

Theou O, Brothers TD, Mitnitski A, Rockwood K (2013) Operationalization of frailty using eight commonly used scales and comparison of their ability to predict all-cause mortality. J Am Geriatr Soc 61:1537–1551

Vidan MT, Sanches E, Alonso M et al (2009) An intervention integrated into daily clinical practice reduces the incidence of delirium during hospitalization in elderly patients. J Am Geriatr Soc 57:2029–2036

Watne LO, Torbergsen AC, Conroy S, Engedal K, Frihagen F, Hjorthaug GA, Juliebo V, Raeder J, Saltvedt I, Skovlund E, Wyller TB (2014) The effect of a pre- and post-operative orthogeriatric service on cognitive function in patients with hip fracture: randomized controlled trial (Oslo Orthogeriatric Trial). BMC Med 12:63

Wong KS, Ryan DP, Liu BA (2014) A system-wide analysis using a senior-friendly hospital framework identifies current practices and opportunities for improvement in the care of hospitalized older adults. J Am Geriatr Soc 62:2163–2170

Young J, Murthy L, Westby M (2010) Diagnosis, prevention and management of delirium: summary of NICE guidance. BMJ 341:c3704

# Case Vignettes

# 11

Pinar Soysal

## 11.1 Case 1

### 11.1.1 Hypoactive Delirium Caused by Pulmonary Embolus in an Elderly Patient

An 87-year-old female patient was brought to the geriatric department because of forgetfulness (not recognizing her children), being introverted, distractibility, indifference to the environment, lack of appetite, refusal of medicines given, and hallucinations such as seeing her deceased husband in the room for the last 2 days. The patient had no known chronic or cognitive deficiency. The physical showed a heart rate of 102 bpm, breath rate of 18 per minute, and a body temperature of 37.4 °C. All systemic exams were found to be normal. Assessment of mental condition revealed cognitive and perception problems with memory and orientation disturbances. The psychomotor activity was declined, and the patient gave short answers to the questions during the interview and refused talking. Based on these clinical findings and symptoms, the newly developed clinical picture was thought to be hypoactive delirium, and the patient was admitted to the geriatric clinic.

The immediate work-up following admission revealed a sinus rhythm electrocardiogram with no pathologic characteristics. She had leukocytosis (13,000/μL). The biochemistry showed normal liver, thyroid, and kidney functions with no electrolyte imbalance. The urinalysis showed no evidence of infection. No pneumonic consolidation or effusion was detected on the chest x-ray. The brain tomography ordered to exclude cranial pathology due to acute mental alteration revealed no pathological findings. Sedimentation was 90 mm/h (*N*, <15 mm/h), C-reactive protein was 115 mg/L (*N*, 0.1–8.2 mg/L), and lumbar puncture was performed to exclude aseptic meningitis and encephalitis, which showed normal results. On the fifth day,

P. Soysal, M.D.
Associate Professor, Kayseri Education and Training Hospital, Geriatrics Center, Kayseri, Turkey
e-mail: dr.pinarsoysal@hotmail.com



A.T. Isik, G.T. Grossberg (eds.), *Delirium in Elderly Patients*,
https://doi.org/10.1007/978-3-319-65239-9_11

the patient was persistently encouraged to mobilize because she did not want to get out of the bed and wished to sleep continuously; however she developed exertional dyspnea and syncope. D-Dimer was elevated, so thorax tomography was ordered. Filling defects at the main and segmental branches of pulmonary arteries consistent with embolus were observed on both sides, being more prominent on the right side, and minimal pleural effusion was observed on the left side. Lower extremity venous Doppler ultrasonography findings were consistent with subacute deep vein thrombosis in the left lower extremity. The patient was started enoxaparin sodium (twice daily), and warfarin was added on this treatment on the third day. On the fifth day of anticoagulant therapy, the delirium picture was completely resolved and the patient was discharged consequently. During the outpatient follow-up, warfarin treatment was regulated to maintain an international normalized ratio level of 2.5–3.5 and the patient developed no new delirium attack Soysal and Isik (2014).

### 11.1.2 Conclusions

Hypoactive delirium is the most commonly encountered subtype in the elderly. Unlike the other subtypes, the patients behave as if they are sedatized and do not give harm to self or others around; as a consequence such patients are often unidentified by the clinicians or take a misdiagnosis, such as depression or dementia. As delirium in the elderly may emerge upon simple situations such as untreated urinary system infection, constipation, and pain, it can also develop upon life-threatening conditions such as myocardial infarction or stroke. Rarely, one of the atypical clinical presentations of pulmonary embolus (PE) may be delirium, as mentioned in this case report, and PE should also be investigated in the elderly subject presenting with delirium condition, even in the absence of typical symptoms. In conclusion, while assessing the etiology of delirium, clinicians should remember that one of the acute conditions leading to development of delirium is PE, particularly in elderly Soysal and Isik (2014).

## 11.2 Case 2

### 11.2.1 Mirizzi Syndrome Causing Delirium in an Elderly Patient

The patient was seen in our outpatient geriatric clinic with symptoms of sudden change in mental status, nervousness, abdominal pain especially in the upper right quadrant, decreased appetite, nausea, and vomiting (temperature, 37.7 °C; and respiration, 22 per minute). He also had jaundice in his sclera. Murphy's sign was positive upon abdominal examination. His mental status examination showed he had cognitive and perceptual problems, including memory loss, disorientation, and difficulty with language and speech. In addition, he had psychomotor agitation and irritability. Because the patient had been followed in our clinic for the previous 2 years, we quickly noticed the acute deterioration in his mental status. According to these clinical signs and symptoms, delirium was diagnosed based on the Confusion Assessment Method.

After hospitalization in the intensive care unit, all of the drugs he had been using were discontinued. Laboratory evaluations revealed mild leukocytosis (8780/mL); erythrocyte sedimentation rate of 34 mm/h; serum glucose, 117 mg/mL; blood urea nitrogen, 28 mg/dL; serum creatinine, 1.1 mg/dL; sodium, 143 mM/L; and potassium, 4.2 mM/L. He had jaundice, with a serum total bilirubin level of 4.1 mg/dL (direct, 1.8 mg/dL; indirect, 2.3 mg/dL). Liver function tests were abnormal: aspartate aminotransaminase, 109 U/L; alanine aminotransferase, 218 U/L; alkaline phosphatase, 278 U/L; and gamma-glutamyltransferase, 192 U/L. Abdominal ultrasonography demonstrated hydropic gallbladder and multiple stones fixed in the infundibular area of the gallbladder close to the junction of the cystic duct and the common bile duct. Extrahepatic biliary ducts above the site of the obstruction were also observed to be slightly dilated. Accordingly, the patient was diagnosed to have a Mirizzi syndrome. Considering all the other predisposing and precipitating factors, our patient was eventually diagnosed to have Mirizzi syndrome-induced delirium. Thereafter, we started a gradually increasing dose of haloperidol up to 2 mg intravenous to control his agitation and psychotic symptoms. For treatment and confirmation of the diagnosis, endoscopic retrograde cholangiopancreatography (ERCP) was performed and showed that the contrast uptake was present to the common hepatic duct and that the calculi in the cystic duct were compressing the superior portion of the common bile duct. On the fifth day after papillatomy by ERCP, the patient became mobile with almost completely resolved neuropsychological status. To prevent recurrence of obstructive jaundice and cholangitis, 6 weeks later, an elective cholecystectomy surgery was performed. The diagnosis of Mirizzi syndrome was also confirmed during surgery. He had an uneventful hospital stay of 1 week and was then called for a follow-up visit after 3 months (Bozoglu et al. 2009).

### 11.2.2 Conclusions

It has been reported that the attending physicians do not detect up to 84–95% of the cases because of the clinical condition itself (which may be misinterpreted as depression, dementia, or even the physiological aging process) or the variability of symptoms, as well as the concomitant presence of etiological factors, which may induce confusion and complicate diagnosis. Clinicians must identify the real underlying medical conditions, for example, Mirizzi syndrome as mentioned in this case report.

## 11.3 Case 3

### 11.3.1 Ogilvie's Syndrome Presented with Delirium in an Older Patient with Renal Cell Carcinoma and Multiple Myeloma

A 77-year-old male admitted to the emergency department with symptoms of sudden change in mental status, nervousness, abdominal distention, and no defecation for 3 days. He had hypertension, renal cell carcinoma, and multiple myeloma. On physical examination, although bowel sounds were present, the abdomen was tympanic. In addition, he had cognitive and perceptual problems and was presenting psychomotor agitation and irritability. According to these clinical signs and symptoms, delirium was diagnosed by Confusion Assessment Method. On admission to hospital, blood analyses revealed the following: white blood cell, 10,600/μL; hemoglobin, 10.6 g/dL; glucose, 133 mg/dL; urea, 66 mg/dL; creatinine, 1.6 mg/dL; sodium (Na+), 142 mM/L; potassium (K+), 5.1 mM/L; and ionized calcium, 1.25 mM/L. Plain and upright abdominal radiograph showed a dilated colon. He was hospitalized and nasogastric aspiration was initiated. In order to stabilize the patient, haloperidol of up to 2 mg was started intravenously. He was then supported with intravenous fluids, and a rectal tube was inserted. At the same time, he was placed in the prone position. Six hours later, although psychotic symptoms were under control, decompression was not achieved. Neostigmine (1.5 mg) infusion was started, and defecation was achieved. The following day, neostigmine infusion was repeated. On the fourth day of hospitalization, colonic decompression was completely achieved and the patient was discharged.

### 11.3.2 Conclusions

Delirium is often not recognized by health professionals, either due to the clinical condition itself or due to the variability of symptoms, as well as to the concomitance of etiologic factors. To avoid unnecessary interventions, comprehensive geriatric assessment should be recommended for the optimum management of older patients, as in this case (Isik et al. 2010).

## 11.4 Case 4

### 11.4.1 Non-pharmacological Approaches Might Reduce the Incidence, Duration, and Total Episodes of Delirium

During the course of rehabilitation, a 78-year-old man presented with immobilization and deconditioning that began 15 days after surgery for a left-sided total hip arthroplasty. His relatives also revealed that he had suffered a severe depressive mood, including fear of falling, within the past 3–4 days. Episodes of agitation, sleep disturbance, decreased attention, confusion, and hallucinations, especially at night, were also present. Accordingly, his rehabilitation process had been affected unfavorably. The medical history was otherwise unremarkable. Results from a cognitive evaluation of the patient (during the day) were normal except for disorientation in regard to time. Physical examination revealed painful and limited movement of the left hip joint. His neurological evaluation was unremarkable. Laboratory evaluations—including a complete blood count and liver and renal function tests, erythrocyte sedimentation rate, urine analysis, and urine, blood, and stool cultures—were all normal. Overall, the patient was diagnosed as having delirium. After reassuring the patient and relatives about the diagnosis, the physician began treatment with trazodone 50 mg/day and recommended modifying the room to provide sufficient day-night lighting, installing a calendar and clock to help the patient be aware of time, having family photographs available to the patient for personal orientation, and removing extra objects from the room to decrease disturbing sensory input. On the seventh day of the control visit, the patient was observed to improve significantly (with increased voluntary participation during rehabilitation and decreased agitation). On day 35 of his hospital stay after complete recovery, the patient was discharged. He could ambulate independently by using a walker and trazodone treatment was stopped (Tekin et al. 2011).

### 11.4.2 Conclusion

Since non-pharmacological approaches including orientation to the surroundings and care team members, uninterrupted nighttime, sleep, early mobilization, and optimum vision and hearing might reduce the incidence, duration, and total episodes of delirium, they should be performed on all the patients who have great risks for delirium.

## References

Bozoglu E, Isik AT, Comert B et al (2009) Mirizzi syndrome causing delirium in an elderly patient. J Am Geriatr Soc 57(2):362–364

Isik AT, Aydin S, Bozoglu E (2010) Ogilvie's syndrome presented with delirium in an older patient with renal cell carcinoma and multiple myeloma. Turk J Gastroenterol 21(2):192–193

Soysal P, Isik AT (2014) Hypoactive delirium caused by pulmonary embolus in an elderly adult. J Am Geriatr Soc 62(3):586–587. https://doi.org/10.1111/jgs.12720

Tekin L, Ozcakar L, Isik AT (2011) Delirium: a critical diagnosis for every member of the rehabilitation team. Rehabil Nurs 36(5):214–215

# Correction to: Delirium in Elderly Patients

## Correction to: A.T. Isik, G.T. Grossberg (eds.), Delirium in Elderly Patients https://doi.org/10.1007/978-3-319-65239-9

The Appendix "Delirium Assessment Instruments" was missed and it has been included in the backmatter of the book.

The updated online version of this book can be found at https://doi.org/10.1007/978-3-319-65239-9

A. T. Isik (✉)
Department of Geriatric Medicine, Dokuz Eylul University, School of Medicine, Izmir, Turkey

G. T. Grossberg
Department of Neurology and Psychiatry, Saint Louis University, School of Medicine, St. Louis, MO, USA


A. T. Isik, G. T. Grossberg (eds.), *Delirium in Elderly Patients*,
https://doi.org/10.1007/978-3-319-65239-9_12

# Appendix: Delirium Assessment Instruments

## The Confusion Assessment Method (CAM)

| | |
|---|---|
| **The diagnosis of delirium by CAM requires the presence of BOTH features A and B** | |
| **A.** | **Acute onset and Fluctuating course**<br>Is there evidence of an acute change in mental status from patient baseline? Does the abnormal behavior:<br>– Come and go?<br>– Fluctuate during the day?<br>– Increase/decrease in severity? |
| **B.** | **Inattention**<br>Does the patient:<br>– Have difficulty focusing attention?<br>– Become easily distracted?<br>– Have difficulty keeping track of what is said? |
| **AND the presence of EITHER feature C or D** | |
| **C.** | **Disorganized thinking**<br>Is the patient's thinking<br>– Disorganized<br>– Incoherent<br>For example does the patient have<br>– Rambling speech/irrelevant conversation?<br>– Unpredictable switching of subjects?<br>– Unclear or illogical flow of ideas? |
| **D.** | **Altered level of consciousness**<br>Overall, what is the patient's level of consciousness:<br>– Alert (normal)<br>– Vigilant (hyper-alert)<br>– Lethargic (drowsy but easily roused)<br>– Stupor (difficult to rouse)<br>– Comatose (unrousable) |



A. T. Isik, G. T. Grossberg (eds.), *Delirium in Elderly Patients*,
https://doi.org/10.1007/978-3-319-65239-9

**References**

Inouye SK, vanDyck CH, Alessi CA, Balkin S, Siegal AP, Horwitz RI (1990) Clarifying confusion: the confusion assessment method. A new method for detection of delirium. Ann Intern Med 113:941–948

Inouye SK, Bogardus ST, Charpentier PA, Leo-Summers L, Acampora D, Holford TR, Cooney LM (1999) A multicomponent intervention to prevent delirium in hospitalized older patients. N Engl J Med 340(9):669–676. https://doi.org/10.1056/NEJM199903043400901

## Confusion Assessment Method for the Intensive Care Unit (CAM-ICU)

Features and descriptions (absent/present).

Overall CAMICU assessment (features 1 and 2 and either feature 3 or 4; (yes/no).

1. **Acute onset or fluctuating course**
   A. Is there evidence of an acute change in mental status from the baseline?
   B. Or did the (abnormal) behavior fluctuate during the past 24 h, that is, tend to come and go to increase and decrease in severity as evidenced by fluctations on the Richmond Agitation Sedation Scale or the Glascow Coma Scale?
2. **Inattention**
   Did the patient have difficulty focusing attention as evidenced by a score of fewer than eight correct answers on either the visual or auditory components of the Attention Screening Examination?
3. **Disorganized thinking**
   Is there evidence of disorganized or incoherent thinking as evidenced by incorrect answers to three or more of the four questions and inability to follow the commands?
   Questions
   1. Will a stone float on water?
   2. Are there fish in the sea?
   3. Does 1 pound weigh more than 2 pounds?
   4. Can you use a hammer to pound a nail?

   Commands
   1. Are you having unclear thinking?
   2. Hold up this many fingers (examiner holds two fingers in front of the patient).
   3. Now do the same thing with the other hand (without holding the two fingers in front of the patient).

      (If the patient is already extubated from the ventilator, determine whether the patient's thinking is disorganized or incoherent, such as rambling or irrelevant conversation, unclear or illogical flow of ideas, or unpredictable switching from subject to subject.)

4. Altered level of consciousness Is the patient's level of consciousness anything other than alert, such as being vigilant or lethargic or in a stupor, or coma?
   **Alert:** spontaneously fully aware of environment and interacts appropriately.
   **Vigilant:** hyperalert. Lethargic drowsy but easily aroused, unaware of some elements in the environment or not spontaneously interacting with the interviewer; becomes fully aware and appropriately interactive when prodded minimally.
   **Stupor:** difficult to arouse, unaware of some or all elements in the environment or not spontaneously interacting with the interviewer; becomes incompletely aware when prodded strongly; can be aroused only by vigorous and repeated stimuli and as soon as the stimulus ceases, stuporous subject lapses back into unresponsive state.
   **Coma:** unarousable, unaware of all elements in the environment with no spontaneous interaction or awareness of the interviewer so that the interview is impossible even with maximal prodding.

**Reference**

Ely EW, Inouye SK, Bernand GR, Gordon S, Francis J, May L, et al (2001) Delirium in mechanically ventilated patients: validity and reliability of the confusion assessment method for the intensive care unit (CAM-ICU). J Am Med Assoc 286(21):2703–2710. Retrieved from http://cat.inist.fr/?aModele=afficheN&cpsidt=13531387

## Drugs Highly Associated with Delirium

| | |
|---|---|
| **High risk** | • Centrally acting agents |
| | • Antiparkinsonian agents (particularly anticholinergic agents) |
| | • Antidepressants (particularly anticholinergic agents) |
| | • Benzodiazepines |
| | • Opioid analgesics |
| | • Corticosteroids |
| | • Lithium |
| **Medium risk** | • Nonsteroidal anti-inflammatory drugs |
| | • Antiarrhythmics (highest risk with lidocaine) |
| | • Antipsychotics (particularly sedating agents) |
| | • $\beta$-Blockers |
| | • $\alpha$-Blockers |
| | • Digoxin |
| | • Postganglionic sympathetic blockers |
| **Low risk** | • Anticonvulsants |
| | • Antiasthmatics (highest risk with aminophylline; lowest risk with inhaled agents) |
| | • Antibacterials |
| | • ACE inhibitors |
| | • Calcium channel antagonists |
| | • Diuretics |
| | • $H_2$-Antagonists |

**References**

Bowen JD, Larson EB (1993) Drug-induced cognitive impairment. Defining the problem and finding the solutions. Drugs Aging 3(4):349–357

Maldonado JR (2008) Pathoetiological model of delirium: comprehensive understanding of the neurobiology of delirium and an evidence-based approach to prevention and treatment. Crit Care Clin 24:789–856

# Index




A.T. Isik, G.T. Grossberg (eds.), *Delirium in Elderly Patients*,
https://doi.org/10.1007/978-3-319-65239-9

MIX
Papier aus verantwortungsvollen Quellen
Paper from responsible sources
FSC® C105338

If you have any concerns about our products,
you can contact us on
**ProductSafety@springernature.com**

In case Publisher is established outside the EU,
the EU authorized representative is:
**Springer Nature Customer Service Center GmbH**
**Europaplatz 3, 69115 Heidelberg, Germany**

Printed by Libri Plureos GmbH
in Hamburg, Germany